LASER DISOBSTRUCTION AND LASER–ASSISTED BALLOON ANGIOPLASTY

Teruo Matsumoto, M.D., Ph.D.
Professor and Director
Vascular and Laser Surgery
Hahnemann University School of Medicine

Joaquin Sariego, M.D.
Assistant Professor and Director
Endoscopic Surgery
Hahnemann University School of Medicine

Chiaki Sano, M.D., Ph.D.
Assistant Professor
Second Department of Surgery
Hahnemann University School of Medicine

Ryunosuke Kumashiro, M.D., Ph.D.
Associate Professor
Second Department of Surgery
Fukuoka University, Japan

Morris D. Kerstein, M.D.
Professor and Chairman
Department of Surgery
Hahnemann University School of Medicine

Takeshi Okamura, M.D., Ph.D.
Assistant Professor
Department of Surgery
Sangyo School of Medicine, Japan

Ishiyaku EuroAmerica, Inc.
St. Louis • Tokyo

Book Editor: Gregory Hacke, D.C.

FIRST EDITION

Ishiyaku EuroAmerica, Inc.
716 Hanley Industrial Court, St. Louis, Missouri 63144

Library of Congress Catalogue Number 91-070473

Teruo Matsumoto
Laser Disobstruction and Laser-Assisted Balloon Angioplasty: A Color Atlas

ISBN 0-912791-66-7

Ishiyaku EuroAmerica, Inc.
St. Louis • Tokyo

Composition by HiTec Typeset, Columbia, Missouri
Printed and bound by: Espaxs, S.A. Publicaciones Médicas, Rosselló, 132, 08036 Barcelona, Spain

TABLE OF CONTENTS

1. GENERAL CONSIDERATIONS **1**
Introduction **1**
Laser physics **2**
Laser probes; Structure and Types **8**
Equipment **10**
Laser safety **16**

2. LASER SYSTEMS AND THEIR OPERATION **19**

3. THE PERCUTANEOUS APPROACH **29**
Indications **29**
Procedures **30**
Complications **43**

4. THE SURGICAL APPROACH **45**
Indications **45**
Procedures **46**
Complications **59**

5. LASER-ASSISTED BALLOON ANGIOPLASTY (LABA) **61**
Indications **61**
Procedure **62**
Complications **65**

6. LASER ANGIOPLASTY (LA) **67**
Indications **68**
Procedure **68**
Complications **70**

7. LASER COMPLICATIONS **71**
Acute Complications **71**
Intima dissection **71**
Arterial wall perforation **72**
Embolization in distal artery **73**
Chronic Complications **73**
Thrombus formation **73**
Pseudoaneurysm formation **73**

8. LIMITATIONS OF LASER TREATMENT **75**
Extent of lesion **75**
Characteristics of lesion **76**

9. SELECTED CASE STUDIES **77**
Tight stenosis of SFA **77**
Segmental occlusion of SFA **79**
Total length occlusion of SFA **82**
Occlusive lesion of PA **84**
Combined lesions **85**
Summary **88**
References **89**
Appendix **95**

Chapter 1

GENERAL CONSIDERATIONS

Introduction

The theoretical concept of the laser was proposed by Einstein in 1917,[1] but 50 years passed before the first generating laser was designed.[2,3] Since then the laser has been widely applied in medicine,[4-26] and recently lasers have been used for the treatment of cancer.[27-52] Lasers are also being used experimentally[53-55] as well as clinically in the ablation of atheromatous plaques in peripheral and coronary arterial occlusive diseases.[56-73] Acceptable clinical results in laser angioplasty used for ischemic limb salvage have also encouraged its application in such lesions.[62-67,69-73] Expanding future laser applications, however, requires the development of appropriate indications. Laser angioplasty will never replace bypass surgery, but laser treatment may be useful for patients having incapacitating intermittent claudication, rest pain or tissue loss in certain conditions in conjunction or combination with reconstructive surgery.

We once used the Argon laser, with its low-energy (15 watts) and small diameter probes (2.0 mm), in limited applications. Now the YAG laser, with its higher-energy (60 watts) and larger-diameter probes (2.5, 3.5, 4.2 and 5.0 mm), has replaced the Argon laser. Additional balloon angioplasty is used after recanalization to achieve better arteriographic and clinical results, a procedure which we refer to as Laser-Assisted Balloon Angioplasty or LABA. Compared to bypass surgery, laser surgery, if indicated, affords decreased hospitalization time and reduced postoperative morbidity, although it's durability is yet unknown. A simple percutaneous approach minimizes operative time and patients' discomfort.

Laser applications do have associated complications such as vessel wall perforation, intimal dissection, and thrombosis. Appropriate indications for application and a skilled, trained operating team therefore ensure better surgical results and decreased complications.

Essential equipment, applications, techniques, clinical indications, complications and their management will be considered in this book. Unlike electrocautery, laser energy does not interfere with electrical impulses. Patients with pacemakers or electrocardiogram (ECG) and electroencephalogram (EEG) changes, therefore, can be treated by laser.

Laser Physics

Principles

The laser is an acronym for light amplification by the stimulated emission of radiation, a process that can efficiently transmit energy through an electro-optical device in the form of a concentrated beam of light. The basic principle underlying the laser is that when an atom of a substance in an excited state undergoes a spontaneous decay, it emits a photon. In the laser that photon interacts with another energized atom and stimulates the emission of another photon with precisely the same wave characteristics. Each of these identical photons then further stimulate energized atoms to produce additional identical photons cumulatively. The light waves generated in this way are reflected back and forth repeatedly between mirrors set on either end of the laser chamber. Eventually, the laser beam leaves the chamber through a hole at the center of the partially reflective mirror.[74-77] In surgical applications the beam is carried out to the laser tip by a fiberoptic device (the laser probe).

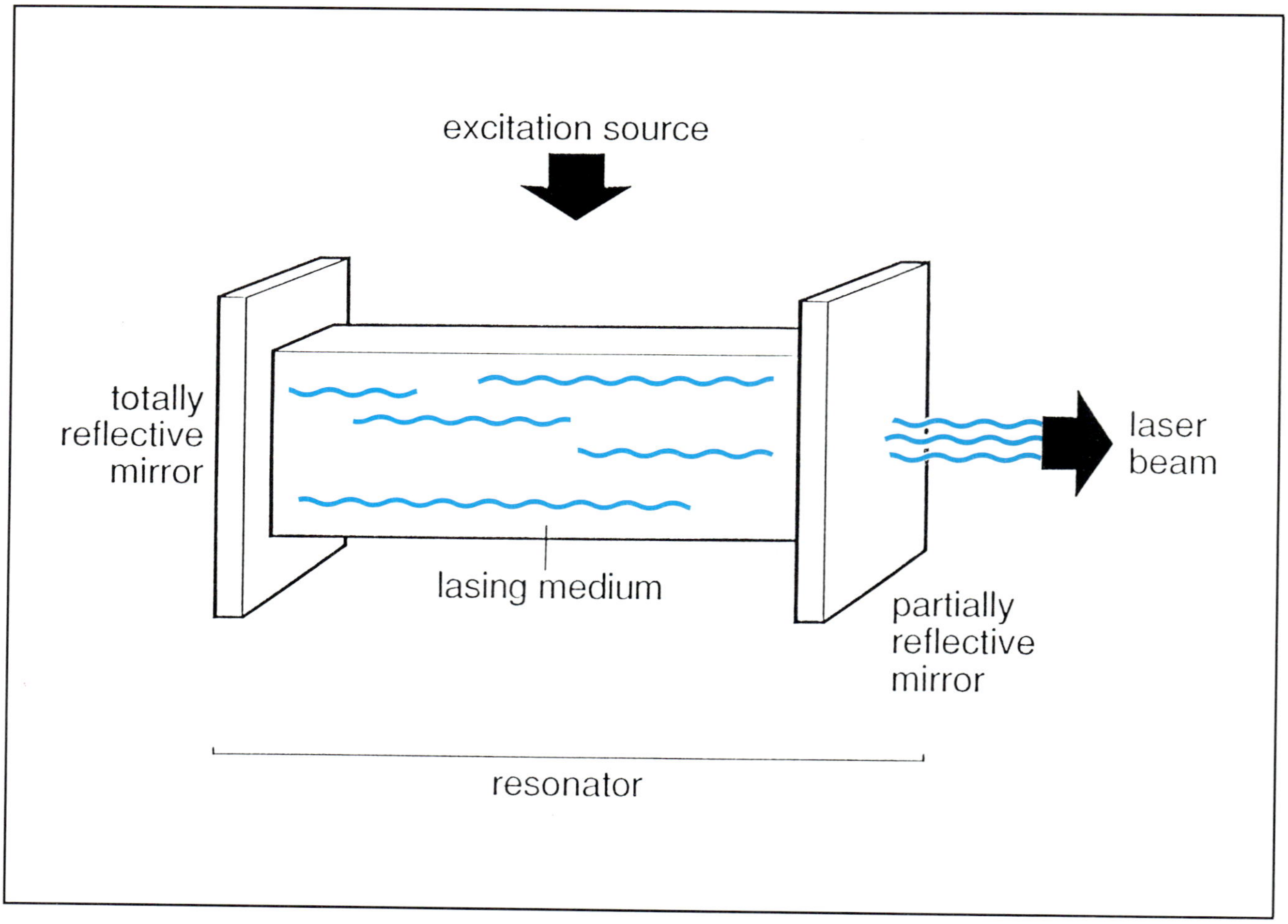

Fig. 1. All laser systems fundamentally consist of three components: 1) a lasing medium (gas, liquid, solid); 2) an excitation source that provides high energy for the medium; and 3) a resonator consisting of a totally reflective mirror and partially reflective mirror.

Basic Laser Properties

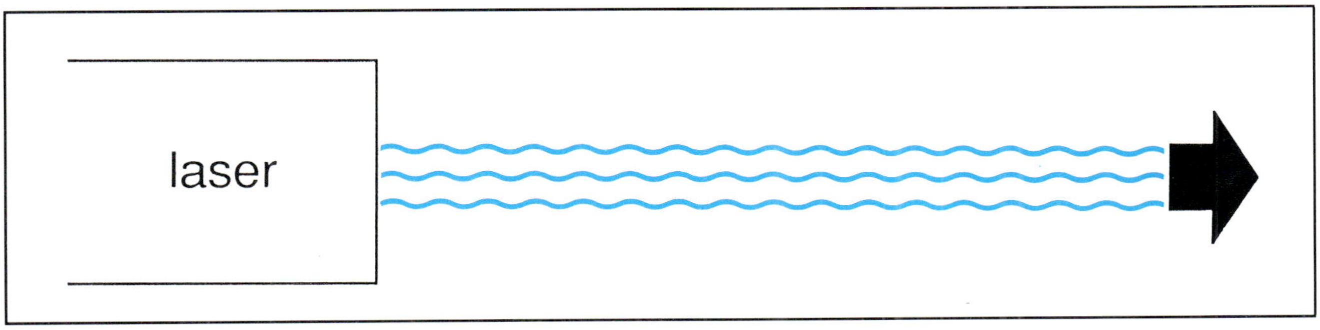

Fig. 2. Laser light has three basic properties: it consists almost exclusively of one wavelength advancing in the same direction (Coherence);

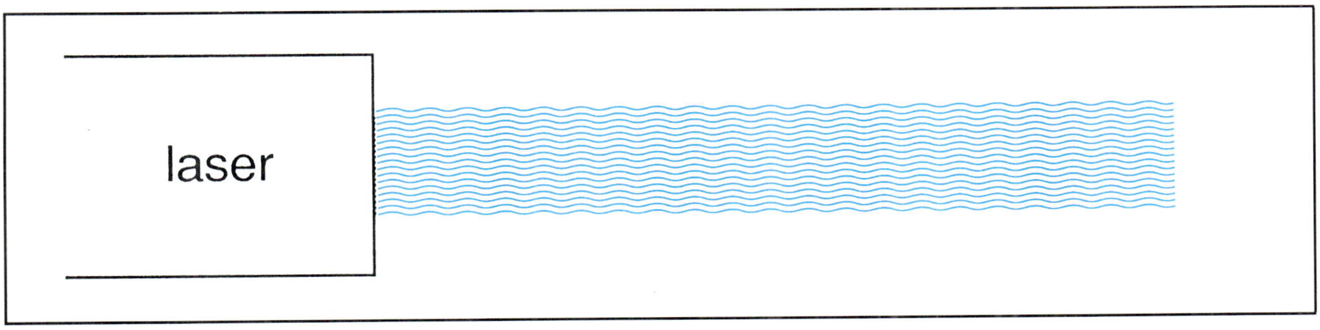

Fig. 3. the light is traveling in a parallel plane with no divergence (Collimation);

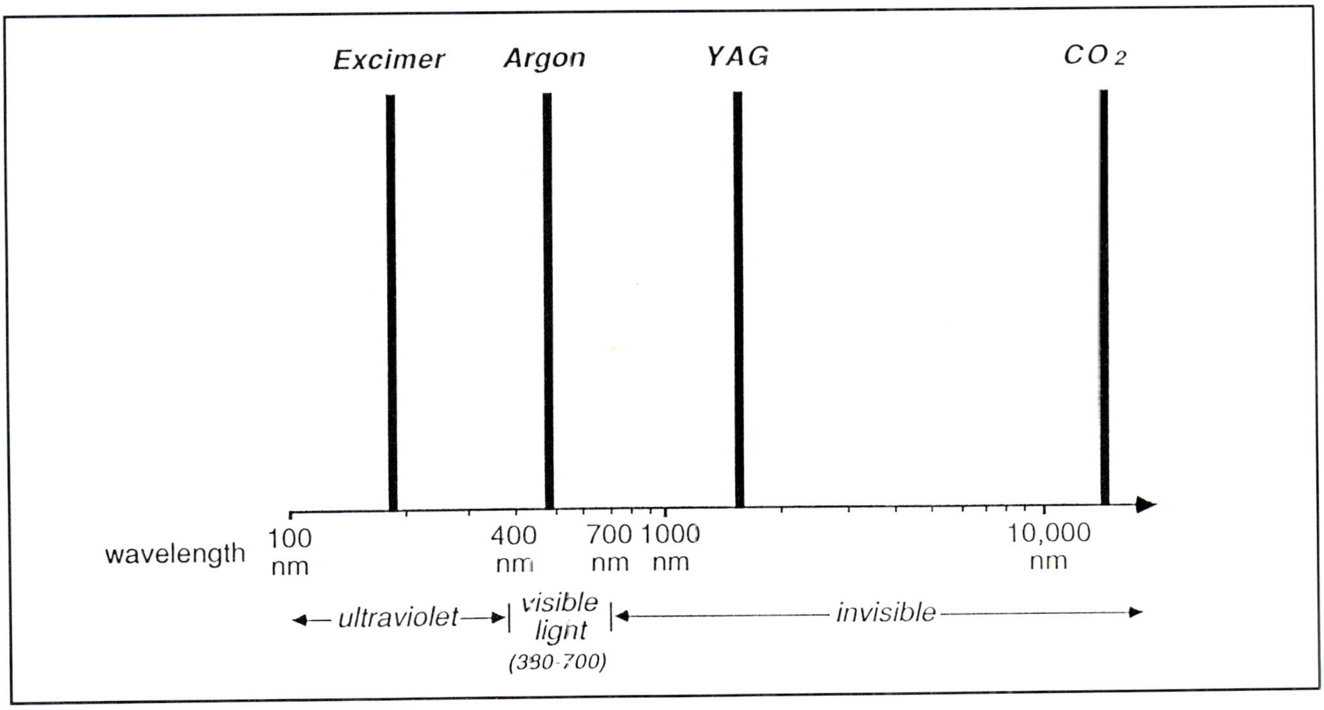

Fig. 4. all laser energy intensifies at one wavelength and barely deviates (Monochromaticity).

Tissue Interaction

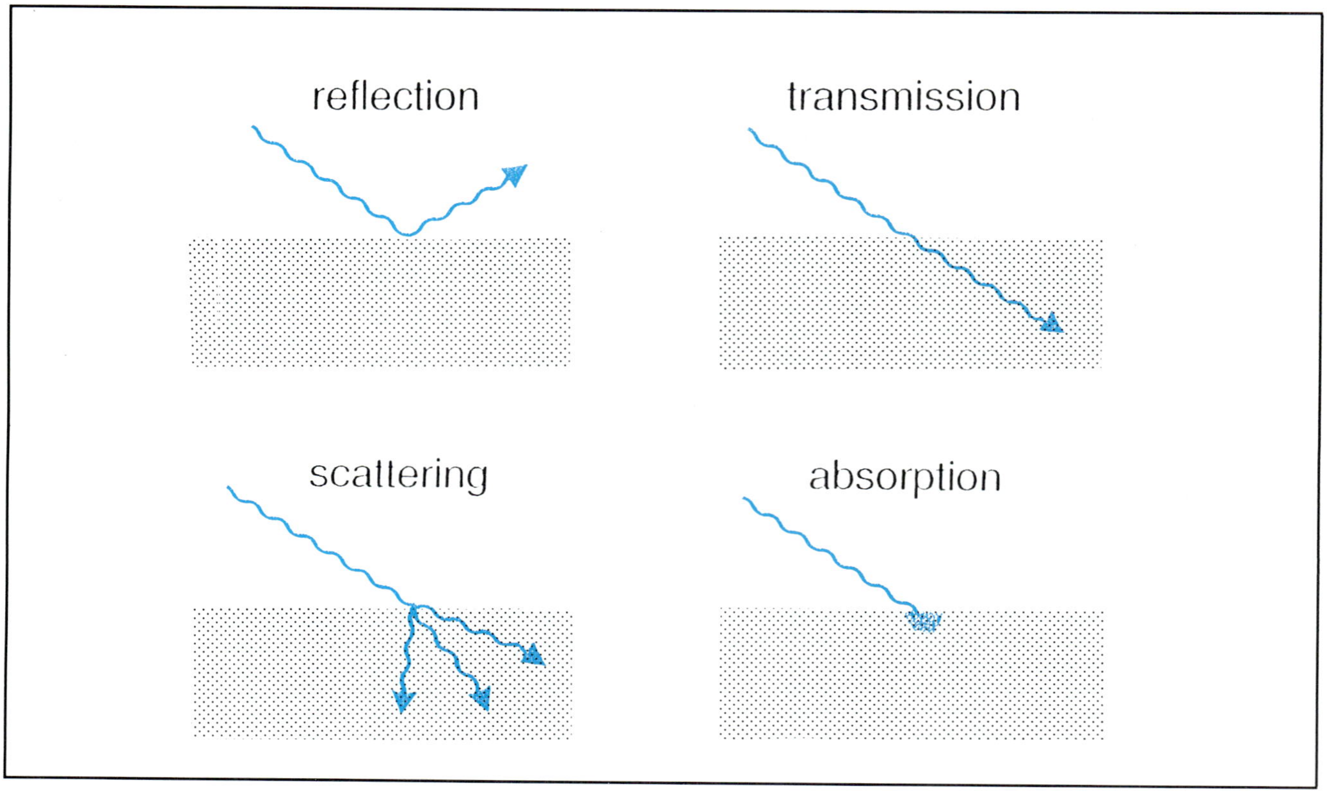

Fig. 5. Laser light has four fundamental interactions with biologic tissue: 1) Reflection, 2) Transmission, 3) Scattering and 4) Absorption. The laser light reflects at the surface of the tissue, transmits through the tissue media, scatters into the tissue and is absorbed by the tissue. In reflection, the tissue is not affected, and in transmission minimal or no change occurs. In scattering, a laser beam is scattered and diffusely absorbed over a wide area weaking its effects. In absorption, however, the effects of the laser beam occur within a limited tissue volume, thus making those effects more pronounced.

Effects of Laser Light (Energy) on Cellular Structures

Cellular degeneration (Coagulation)

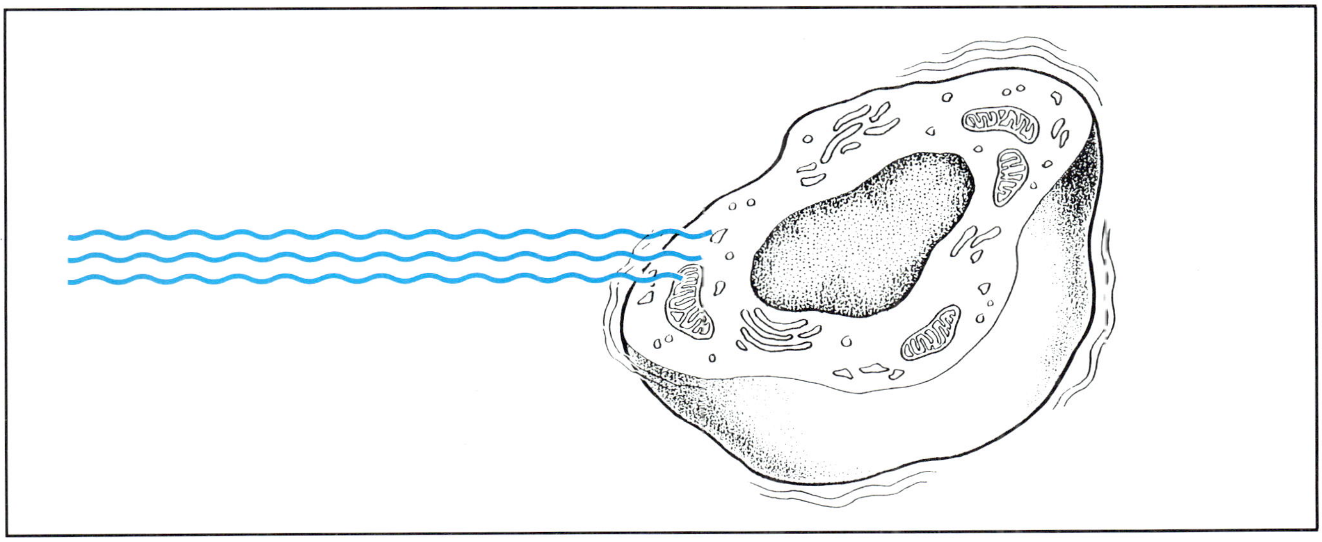

Fig. 6. Upon exposure to laser light, a cell absorbs that light. Consequently, intracellular temperature reaches 60°C and all cellular proteins coagulate. Eventually the cell will degenerate.

Cellular Disruption (Vaporization)

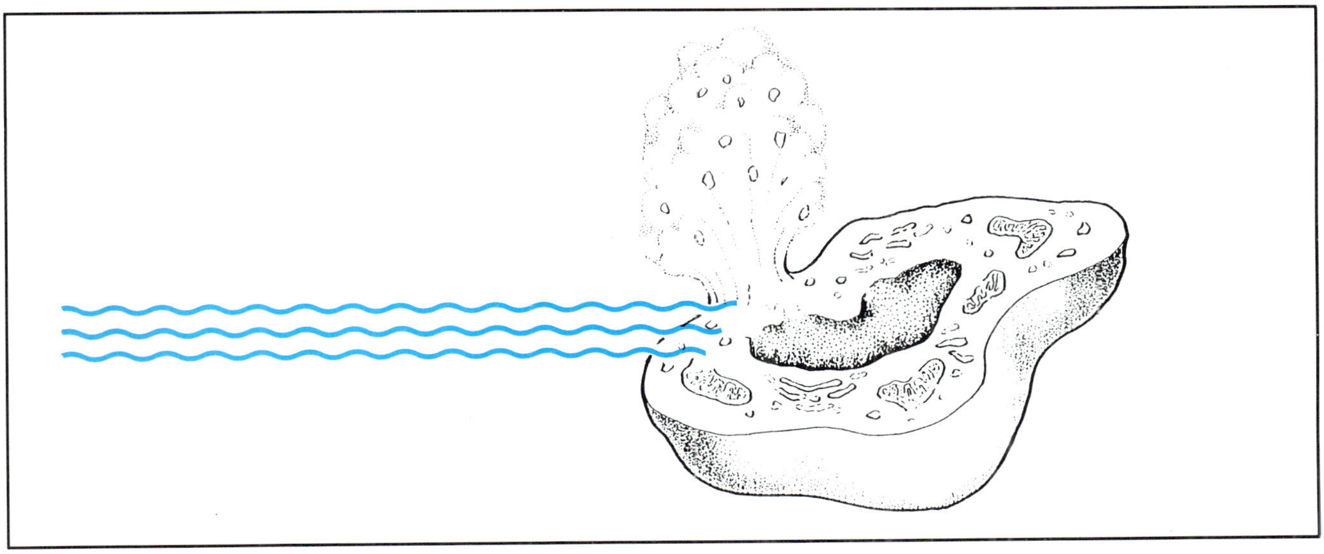

Fig. 7. Cellular water boils when its temperature reaches 100°C after being exposed to laser light. This process ultimately generates steam, which disrupts the cellular wall and explodes the cellular contents.

Cellular destruction (Burning)

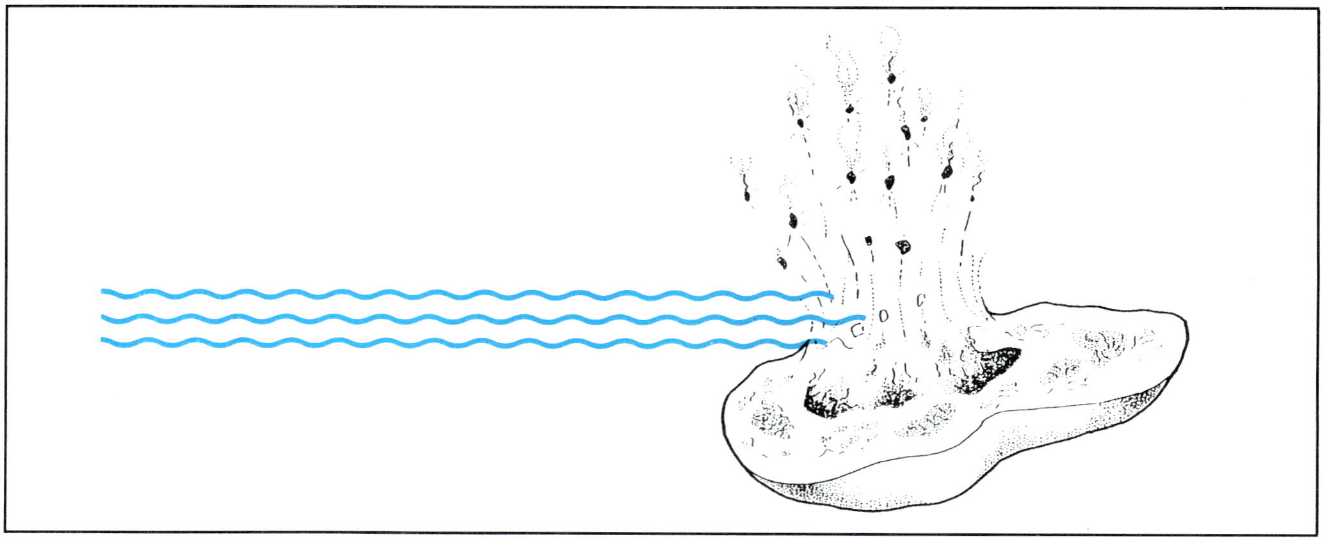

Fig. 8. After cell water evaporation, the temperature of the remaining cellular materials quickly rises with continued use of the laser beam. At 400 - 500°C, all residual cellular materials are charred.

Types of Laser

Several types of lasers are listed according to physical properties. Characteristics of those lasers are shown in Tables 1 and 2.

The carbon dioxide(CO_2, Argon and Neodymium Yttrium Aluminium Garnet (Nd:YAG) laser systems are the most commonly used for therapeutic purposes. The CO_2 laser is invisible (10600-nanometer wavelength, infrared). Its high degree of absorption with limited lateral damage,[78-80] makes it useful as a surgical instrument for cutting tissue.

The Argon laser has a visible blue-green light and easily passes through clear aqueous media. Tissue pigments such as melanin and hemoglobin absorb the Argon laser light, resulting in sufficient localized heat generation to make the Argon laser a highly effective photocoagulator. Retinal disorders[4,6,7,81] and some pigmented lesions of skin such as portwine stains,[82] Nevi aranei[83] and teleangiectasia[84] are, therefore, best treated by applying this principle of selective absorption of the Argon laser light.[85]

The Nd:YAG laser beam is invisible (1064-nanometer wavelength, infrared light) when advancing through clear liquids, but its absorption by tissue is not dependent on color. A power level of 15 to 100 watts will coagulate vessels up to 3 mm in diameter.[86] A high degree of scattering within tissue may affect areas 3 mm from the hitting site. Because of these characteristics, the Nd:YAG laser is useful in tissue coagulation.[87-93]

Table 1. Characteristics of Some Laser Light

Substance	Laser	Wavelength (nanometer)	Color
Gases	Excimer[1]	175-351	Ultraviolet
	Argon	488.0	Blue
		514.5	Green
	Krypton	530.9	Green
		568.2	Yellow
		647.1	Red
	CO_2[2]	10600.0	Infrared
Solids	Nd:YAG[3]	1064.0	Infrared
	Ruby	694.3	Red
Liquid	Rhodamine dye	530-640	Green-Red

[1]Excimer lasers are generated from gas mixtures of halogens (F, Cl, Br) and rare gases (Ar, Kr, Xe).
[2]CO_2: Carbon dioxide
[3]Nd:YAG: Neodymium yttrium aluminium garnet

Table 2. Comparison of CO_2, Argon and Nd:YAG Lasers

	CO_2[1]	Argon	Nd:YAG[2]
Power	0-100 W	0-20 W	0-150 W
Penetration	0.5 mm	1 mm	3 mm
Cutting	Good	Poor	Fair
Coagulation	Poor	Fair	Good
Delivery	Articulated arm	Optical fiber	Optical fiber

[1]CO_2: Carbon dioxide
[2]Nd:YAG: Neodymium yttrium aluminium garnet

The excimer laser, a pulsed gas laser, is generated from a mixture of rare gases (argon, krypton or xenon) and halogens (fluoride, chloride, bromide), which produces high energy ultraviolet light with short wavelength pulses.[94] Different mixtures of those gases produce excimer lasers with different energies and wavelengths (Table 3). Isner et al.[95] revealed that the excimer laser can cut tissues without even histologic evidence of thermal damage and suggested it might possibly facilitate a more benign healing process, a less thrombogenic surface, and better preservation of structural tissue integrity; therefore, it has a potential for application in coronary artery disease.[96]

Laser Probes: Structure and Types

In the beginning, laser probes were non-contact only, but recently contact probes have become available. The latter type of probe is better for cutting and coagulation.

In peripheral vascular surgery, the Argon and YAG lasers are cornmonly used. The Argon laser probe has a tiny aperture at its apex from which 20% of the laser beam is delivered directly to the vascular lesion with 80% of the energy activating the laser tip (Model 780-2.0 Spectraprobe PLR, Trimedyne Inc.).

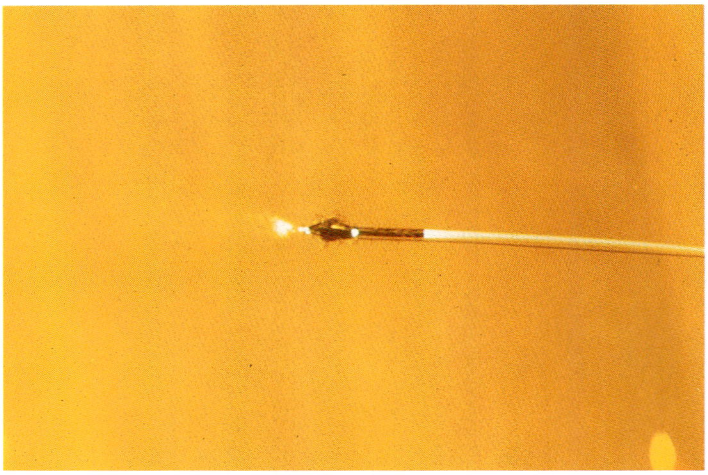

Fig. 9

Table 3. Wavelengths of excimer lasers commonly used.

	Wavelength (Nanometer) Halogens		
Rare gases	**Fluride**	**Chloride**	**Bromide**
Argon	193	175	
Krypton	249	222	
Xenon	351	308	283

Because its energy is limited, the Argon laser's efficacy in severely occlusive lesions is questionable. The YAG laser provides a higher power, but direct application of the beam using a non-contact probe is uncontrollable and detrimental to healthy tissue; therefore, a metal-tipped contact YAG laser probe is now used. With the metal tipped probe, whole laser energy is converted into heat, which can then evaporate atherosclerotic plaque. The diameter of tips available at present are 1.5-mm, 2.0-mm, 2.5-mm (Model 23001), 3.5-mm (Model 23003), 4.2-mm (Model 23004) and 5.0-mm (Model 23006) (Laserprobe-SLR™ Catheter, Trimedyne, Inc.).

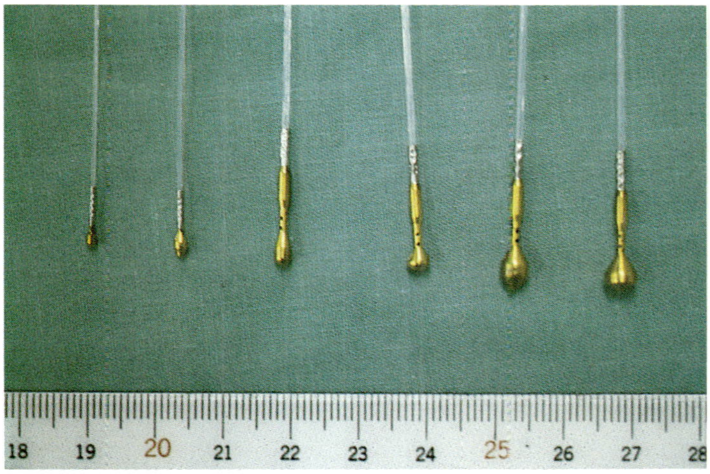

Fig. 10

The 3.5, 4.2 and 5.0 laser tips have small side holes through which a guidewire passes to guide the laser tip.

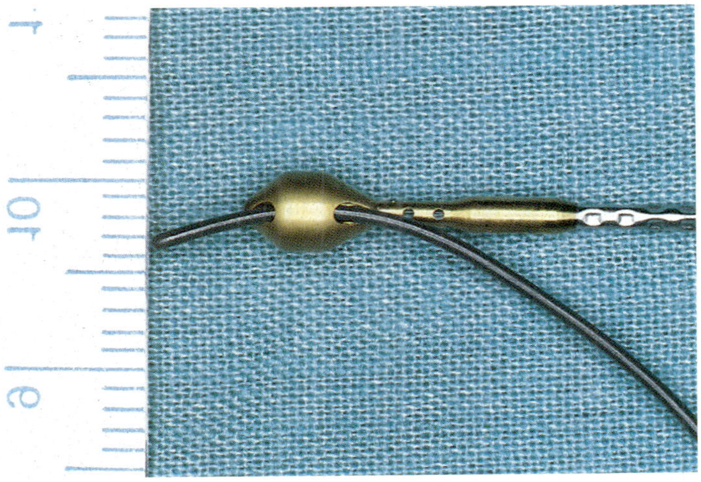

Fig. 11

A newer YAG laser probe has several tiny side apertures that deliver laser energy in direct form (Model 25002, Trimedyne, Inc.).

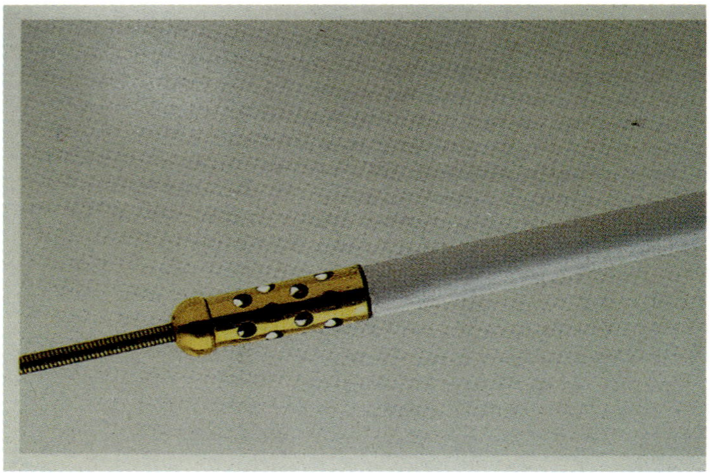

Fig. 12

Equipment

Equipment useful in laser recanalization

1) An 18 gauge needle and a 0.89-mm diameter, 45-cm long J-guidewire (C.R. Bard, Inc.).

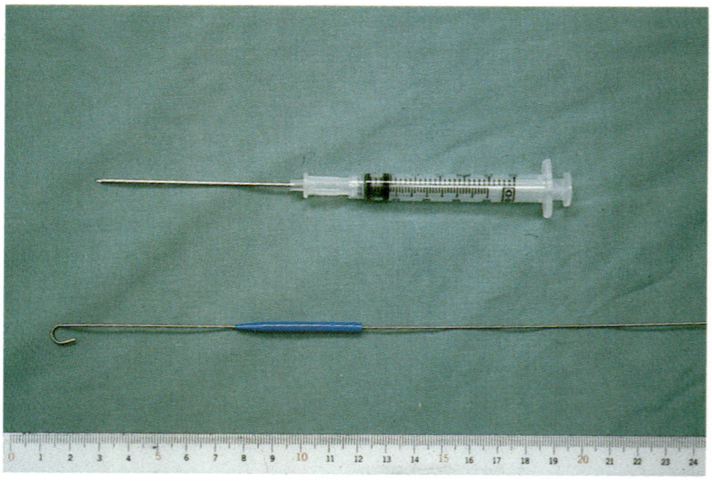

Fig. 13

2) An introducer sheath with side port (No. 8, 9, 12, 14 French) (C.R. Bard, Inc., Teruomo Corp., UMI Corp.).

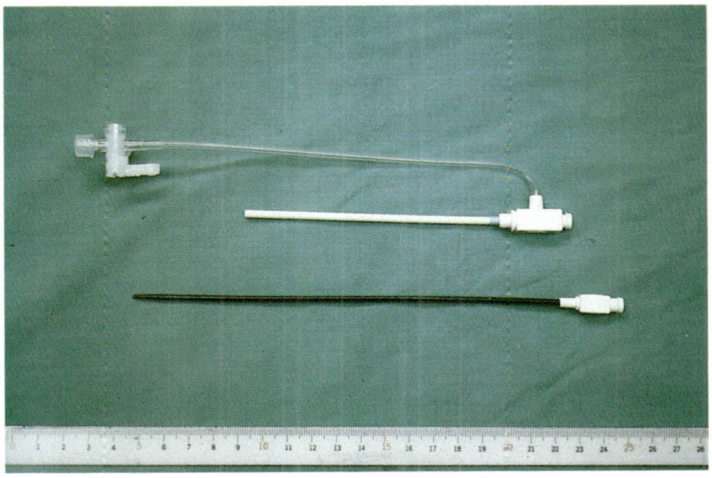

Fig. 14

3) A 0.89-mm diameter, 150-cm long hydrophilic guidewire (Meditech, Inc.).

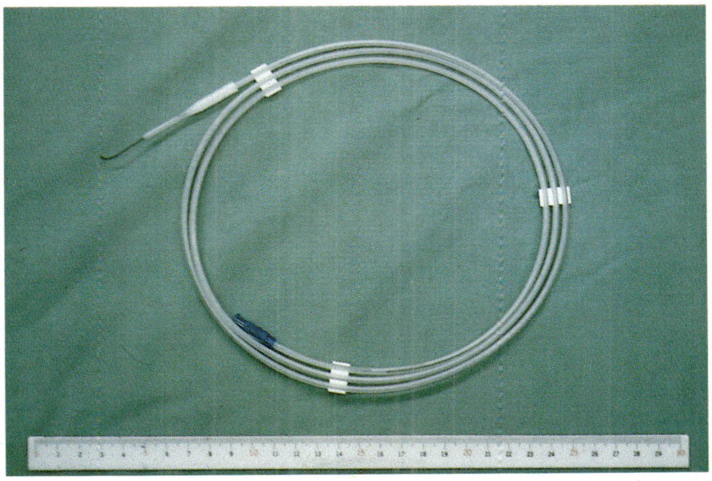

Fig. 15

Equipment facilitating laser recanalization

1) C-arm fluoroscope (General Electric Medical Systems).

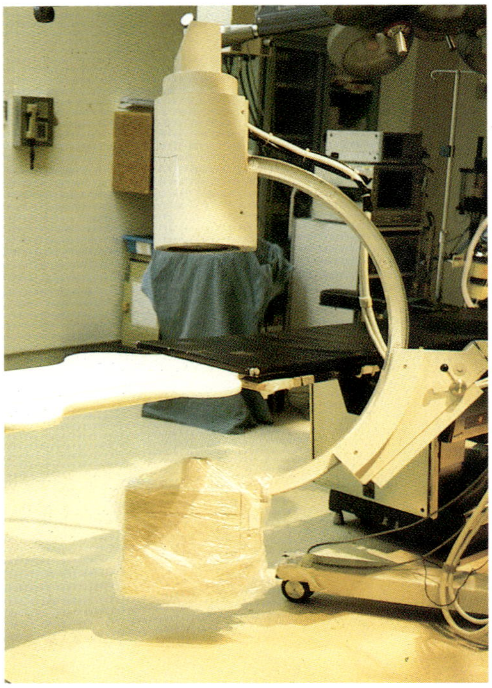

Fig. 16

2) Extension table (Manual table #2080, American Sterilizer Co.) radiolucent for fluoroscopy attachment.

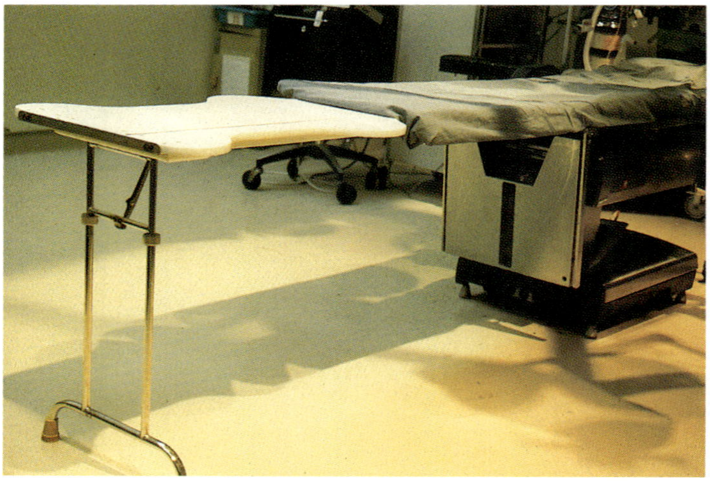

Fig. 17

3) Angioscopes—different types and sizes of angioscopes are available. A 1.4-mm diameter angioscope (PF-14 Ultrathin Fiberscope, Olympus Corp.).

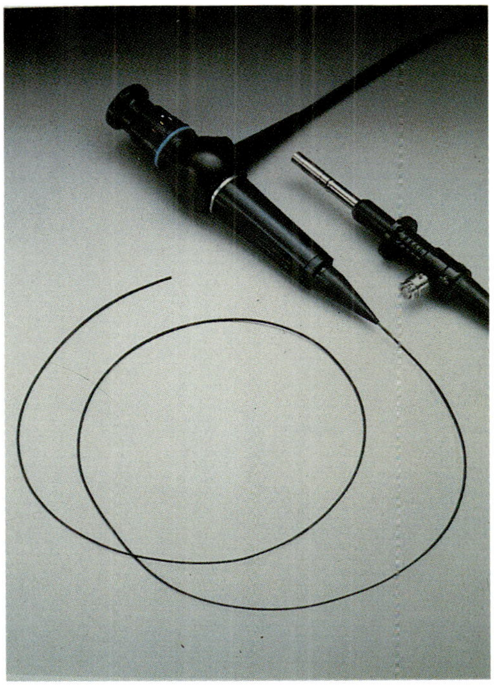

Fig. 18

A 2.0-mm disposable angioscope (Flexible Imaging Catheter #8334, Microvasive).

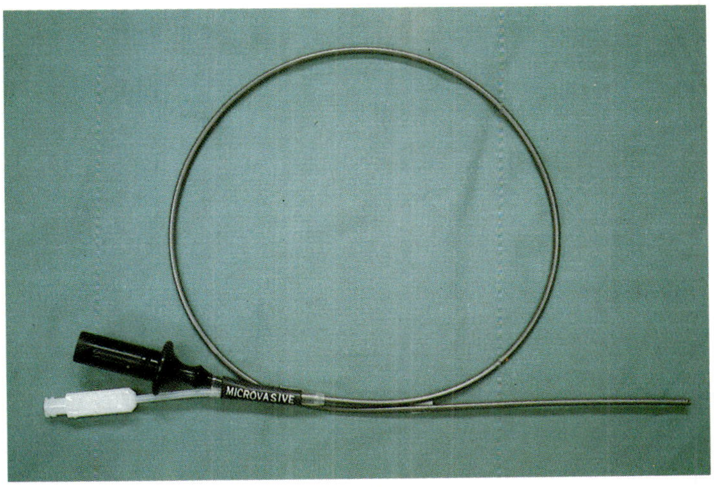

Fig. 19

A 2.5-mm angioscope (Optiscope™ Trimedyne, Inc.). The appropriate size of angioscope, correlating with arterial diameter, should be used to avoid arterial trauma.

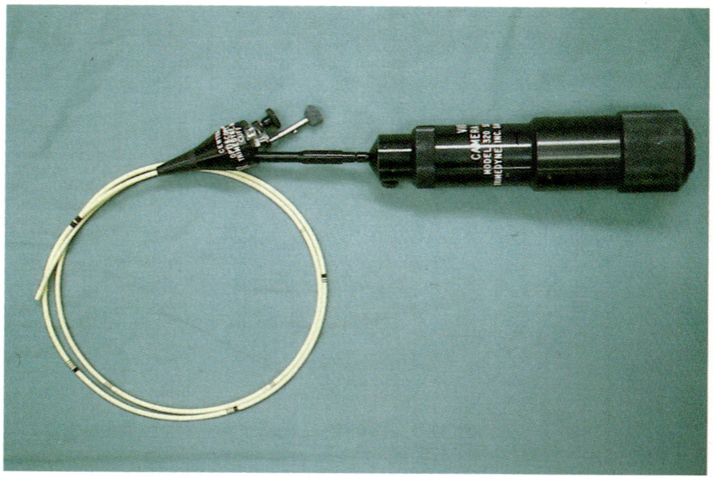

Fig. 20

Additional procedures

1) Gruentzig balloon catheters (2, 3, 4 and 6-mm diameters) are used for dilatation of tibials, popliteal and femoral arteries, respectively (Medi-tech, Inc.). (Fig. 21a and b).

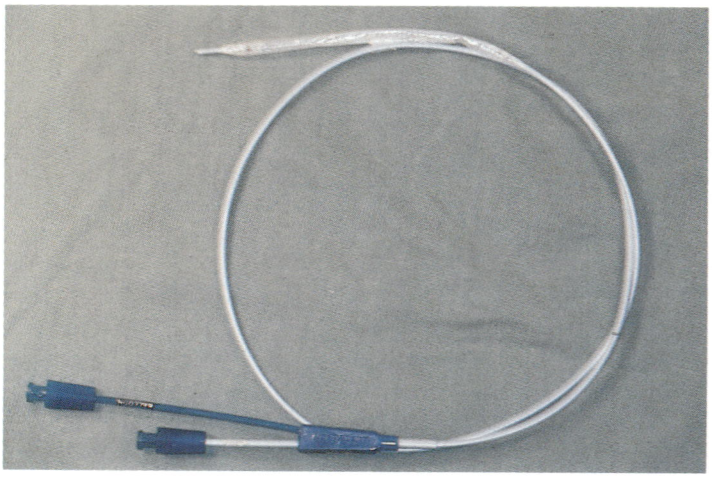

Fig. 21a

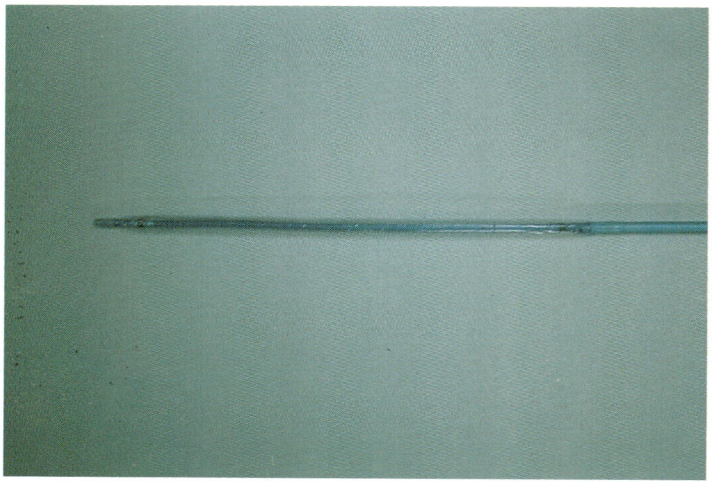

Fig. 21b

2) Olbert balloon catheters (8, 9 and 10-mm diameter, 10-cm length balloon, Meadox Surgimed, Inc.) are used in dilating larger arteries such as the iliac artery and femoral arteries.

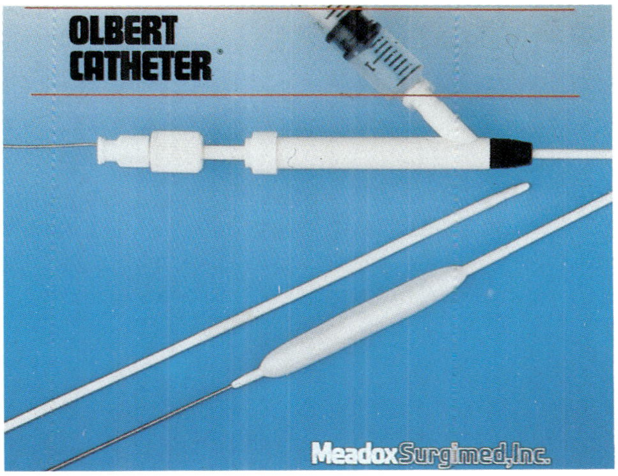

Fig. 22

3) A Leveen inflator (Medi-tech Inc.) used to inflate the balloon. The inflator is calibrated to correlate with Hg pressure.

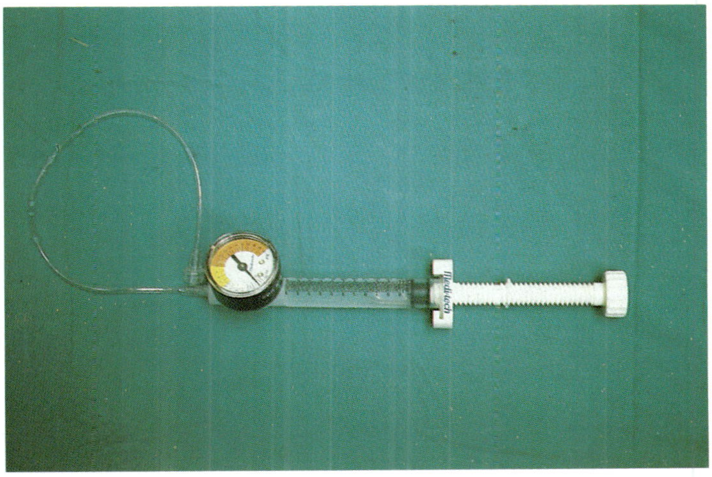

Fig. 23

4) Inflation handle (Meadox Surgimed Inc., Oakland, NJ) increases atmospheric pressure (ATM) by pushing the plunger handle inward. Two red lines on the plunger indicate 10 ATM and 12 ATM at the proximal and distal lines, respectively.

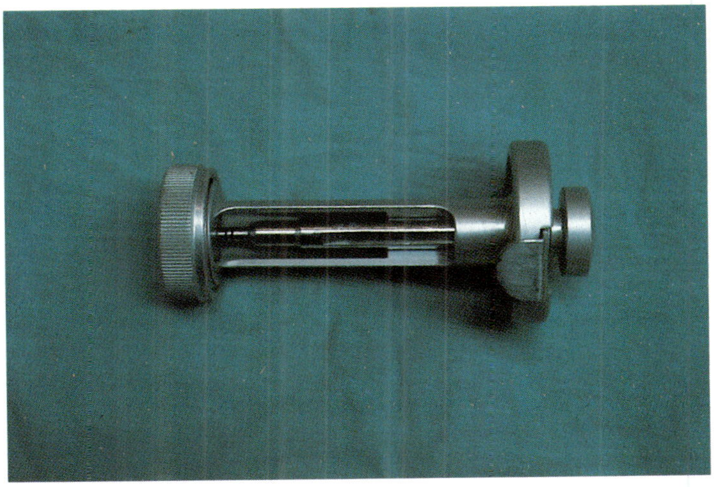

Fig. 24

Laser Safety

National regulating authorities[97-102] classify laser hazards into four different types (Table 4). All class IV lasers should be "key-enabled" to restrict usage.

Staring at a laser beam with the naked eye will cause permanent vision damage. The detrimental effects of lasers include total blindness, skin burns and spontaneous ignition of chemicals or combustible gases.

Table 4. Characteristics of laser hazards

Class I	Power does not exceed eye MPE*	Practically not hazardous to the eye
Class II	Power up to 1 miliwatt, visible laser beam only	Eye can be protected by blink reflex time of 0 to 25 seconds.
Class IIIa	1 to 5 miliwatts for visible radiation	Eye can be protected by blink reflex
IIIb	5 miliwatts to 0.5 watts	Direct viewing hazardous
Class IV	Over 0.5 watts	Extremely hazardous

*Maximum Permissible Exposure

Optical safety considerations

To prevent eye damage, the following safety precautions must be observed. Protective eye glasses MUST BE WORN to filter out the wavelength that emerges extremely to avoid direct laser exposure, and prevent eye injury. Also avoid staring directly into the laser beam.

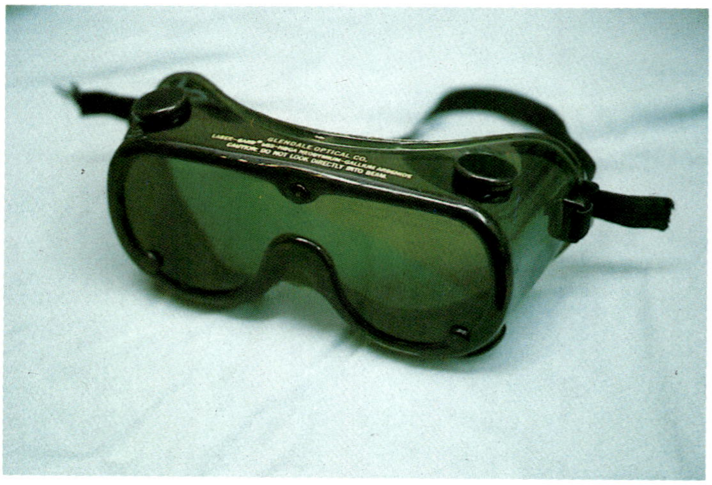

Fig. 25

Electrical safety considerations

High-voltage electricity capable of causing death is used in this system. Extreme caution should be exercised at all times while the system is on. Never work on electrical equipment unless another person familiar with the operations and hazards of the equiqment is nearby and knows first aid. When the situation permits, keep one hand away from the equipment to reduce the hazard of current flowing through vital organs of the body.

Safety consideration

Warning signs

Appropriate warning signs should be placed on every entrance of the operating room.

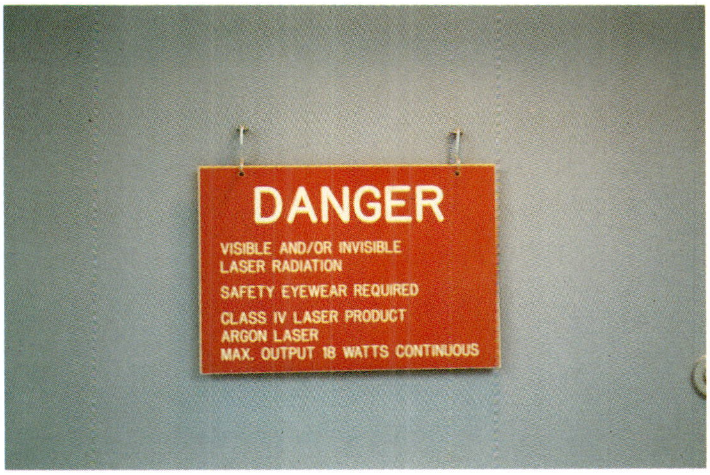
DANGER
VISIBLE AND/OR INVISIBLE
LASER RADIATION
SAFETY EYEWEAR REQUIRED
CLASS IV LASER PRODUCT
ARGON LASER
MAX. OUTPUT 18 WATTS CONTINUOUS

Fig. 26

A warning lamp located at the room entrance should be turned on when the laser is in use.

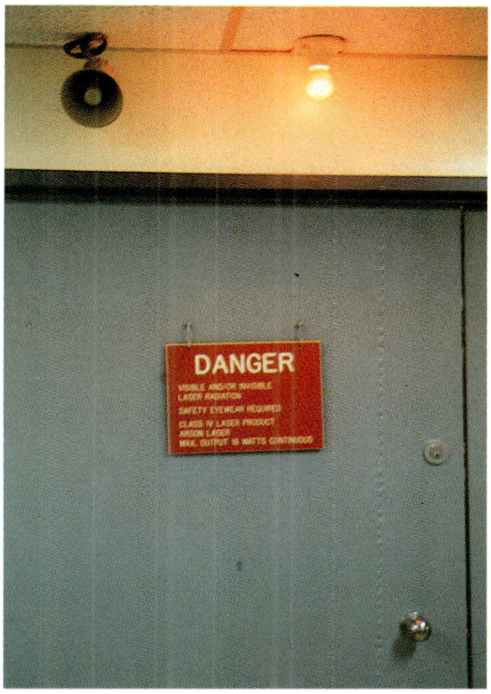
DANGER

Fig. 27

Window covering

All windows must be covered to avoid accidental exposure to outsiders.

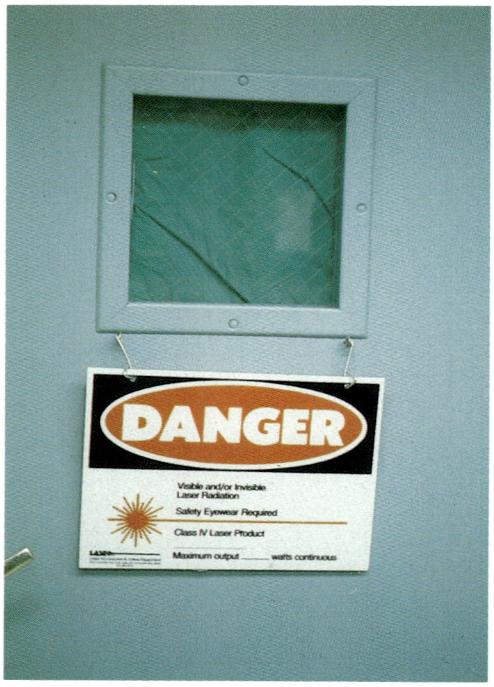
DANGER
Visible and/or Invisible Laser Radiation
Safety Eyewear Required
Class IV Laser Product
Maximum output ____ watts continuous

Fig. 28

Door interlocks

All doors of the operating room should have a lock and should be locked while the laser machine is in use.

Smoke evacuation

The CO_2 laser generates large amounts of smoke and steam. When using it at low energy, the steam has the potential of destroying viable cells. The smoke can cause asphyxiation and poor visualization. The evacuator nozzle, therefore, should be placed as close to the laser handpiece as possible so that the smoke and steam will be completely removed from the surgical field. Compared to the CO_2 laser system, smoke generation in the Argon and YAG laser systems is limited.

Fire safety

A direct beam could cause fire when it is used near flammable materials such as surgical drapes, dressings or alcohol. Laser beam application should be directed at the appropriate site only. Laser-trained staff must be aware of all potential fire hazards and proper response to those situations.

Guidelines for laser use, maintenance and education in Hahnemann University Hospital are shown in Appendix 1.

Chapter 2

LASER SYSTEMS AND THEIR OPERATION

There are several laser systems available for angioplasty (Table 5).

Table 5. Angioplasty Lasers in Clinical Trials (Reprinted with permission: *Laser Medicine & Surgery*. 7:2, 1989)

Manufacturer	Manufacturer	Manufacturer	Manufacturer	Manufacturer	Manufacturer	Manufacturer
Trimedyne Co., Santa Ana, CA (800) 635-5273	GV Medical, Inc., Minneapolis, MN (612) 559-4000	USCI Division, C.R. Bard, Billerica, MA (508) 667-1300 Quantronix Corp. Smithtown, NY (516) 273-6900	MCM Laboratories, Inc., Mountain View, CA (415) 961-2347	Advanced Interventional Systems, Inc. (AIS) Irvine, CA (714) 586-1342	Vaser, Inc., Indianapolis, IN (317) 247-8016 Lambda Physik Acton, MA	Spectranitics Corp., Colorado Springs, (719) 633-8333 CO
System	**System**	**System**	**System**	**System**	**System**	**System**
Optilase 1000 YAG Laser System (60W) Optilase 900 Argon Laser System (12W) LaserProbe PLR peripheral catheter Coronary LaserProbe	Lastac System Argon (18W) Centering Balloon catheter	USCI: Spears Laser Balloon Angioplasty Quantronix; System 1500 Nd:YAG (45W) Laser	MCM Smart Laser: Diagnosis; HeCd 325 UV (8 mw) Treatment; 480 nm pulsed dye (500 ml)	Model 200 308 nm XeCl Excimer	Excimer Laser System 5001 351 nm Excimer VaserGuard catheter tip VaserGuide guidewire	CVX 300 TM 308 nm XeCl Excimer Percutaneous coronary catheter Intraoperative coronary probe
Investigators	**Investigators**	**Investigators**	**Investigators**	**Investigators**	**Investigators**	**Investigators**
Timothy Sanborn, M.D., Mount Sinai Hospital, New York, NY Thomas Linnemeier, M.D., St. Vincent's Medical Center, Indianpolis, IN David Cumberland, M.D., Sheffield, England Richard Leachman, M.D., Texas Heart Institute, Houston, TX	Alberto Foschi, M.D., St. Francis Hospital, Evanston, IL Leonard Nordstrom, M.D., Methodist Hospital, Minneapolis, MN Gene Myers, M.D., Sarasota Memorial Hospital, Sarasota, FL	J. Richard Spears, M.D., Wayne State University, Detroit, MI	Peter Selzer, M.D., Meriter/Madison General Hospital, Madison, WI Frank Veith, M.D., Montifiore Medical Center, New York, NY Marton Leon, M.D., NIH, Bethesda, MD	Frank Litvack, M.D., Cedars-Sinai Medical Center, Los Angeles, CA	John Fehrenbacher, M.D., Methodist Hospital, Indianpolis, IN Donald Schwarten, M.D., St. Vincent's Medical Center, Indianapolis, IN Barry Katzen, M.D., Miami Baptist Hospital, Miami, FL Andrew Cragg, M.D., U. Iowa Hospital, Iowa City, IA	Timothy Sanborn, M.D., Howard Frazier, M.D., Texas Heart Institute, Houston, TX Michael Derns, M.D., Beckmann Laser Institute, California Dr. Bo Johansson, M.D., Upsala Academic Hospital, Upsala, Sweden
Cases	**Cases**	**Cases**	**Cases**	**Cases**	**Cases**	**Cases**
Peripheral: 10,000 Coronary: > 100	Peripheral: 400 Coronary: 25-35	Coronary: > 50	Peripheral: 40 Coronary: 2	Peripheral: 31 Coronary: 2	Coronary: Preclinic R&D	Coronary: 12 intraoperative
FDA Status	**FDA Status**	**FDA Status**	**FDA Status**	**FDA Status**	**FDA Status**	**FDA Status**
Peripheral: PMA Coronary: IDE	Peripheral: PMA Coronary: IDE		Peripheral: IDE Coronary: IDE	Peripheral: IDE Coronary: IDE Phase I	Peripheral: IDE Phase II	Coronary: Phase II intraoperative
Cost	**Cost**	**Cost**	**Cost**	**Cost**	**Cost**	**Cost**
\$96,000 \$400-600 catheter	\$100,000 + \$2,000 procedure	\$100,000-160,000	\$250,000	\$205,000	\$120,000 + \$1,000 disposable catheter	\$180,000

Model 1000 Optilase™ YAG Contact Laser System (Trimedyne, Inc.).

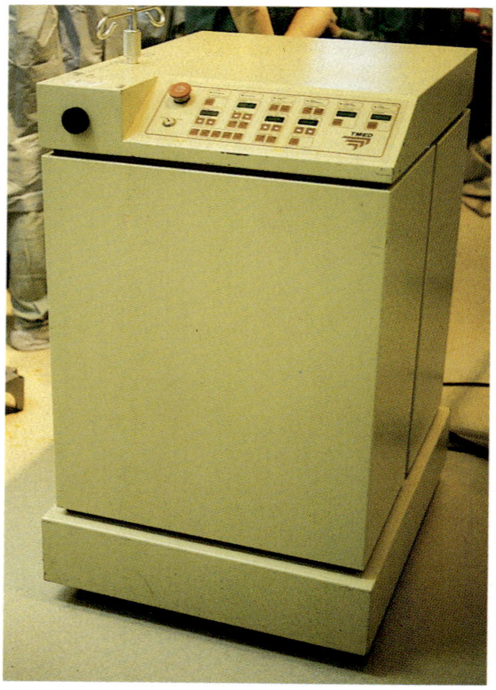

Fig. 29

CL 60 PORTABLE Nd:YAG Laser (Surgical Laser Technologies).

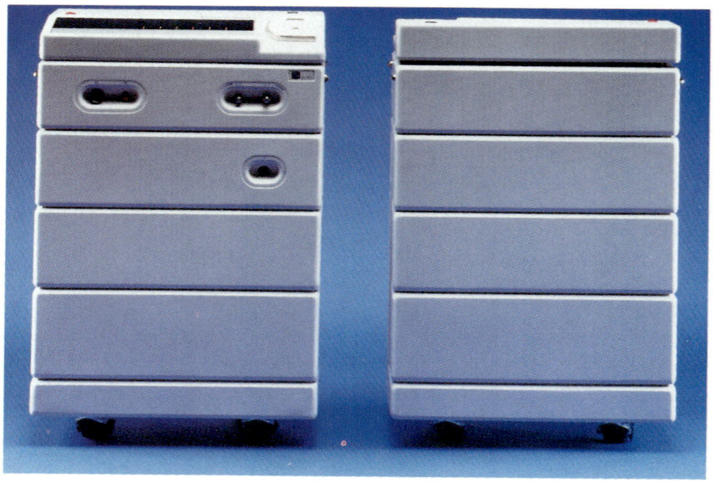

Fig. 30

ExciMed™ UV 300 (Summit Technology, Inc.).

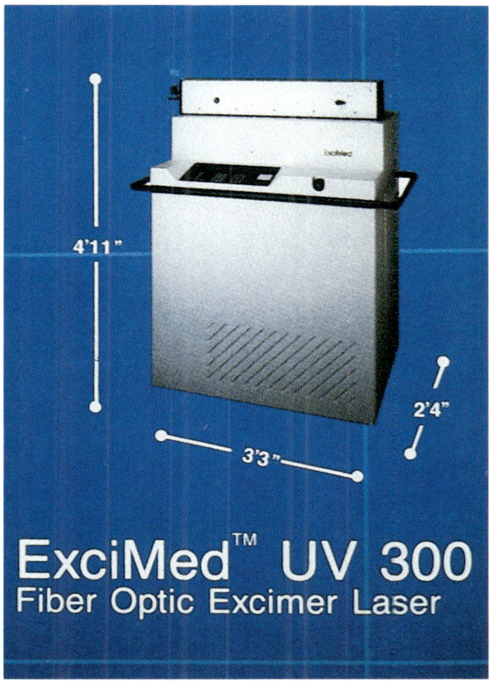

Fig. 31

Operation of Nd:YAG Laser System (Model 1000 Optilase™)

All of the following steps should be exercised sequentially and carefully to ensure proper operation of the laser system. The operation of the Model 1000 Optilase™ is used below as an example, referencing Trimedyne's OPERATION AND SERVICE MANUAL.

Turn on the water valve to make sure that water is circulating through the machine.

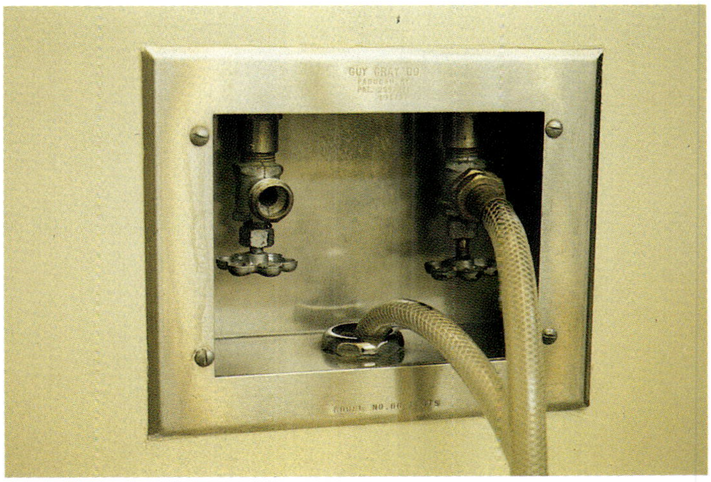

Fig. 32

Connect the power source.

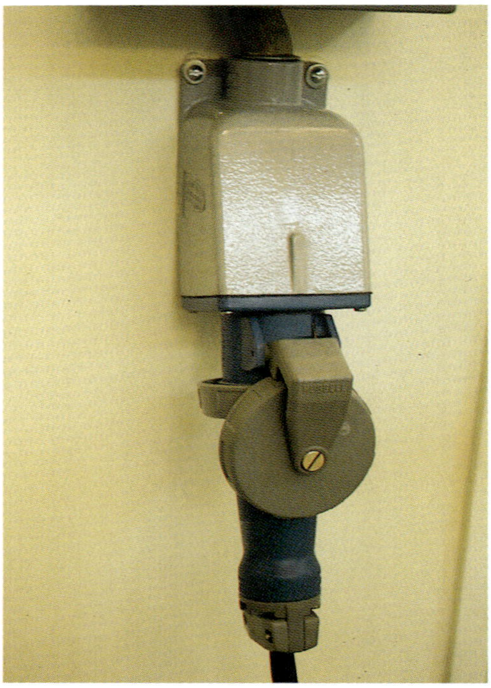

Fig. 33

Turn on the power switch.

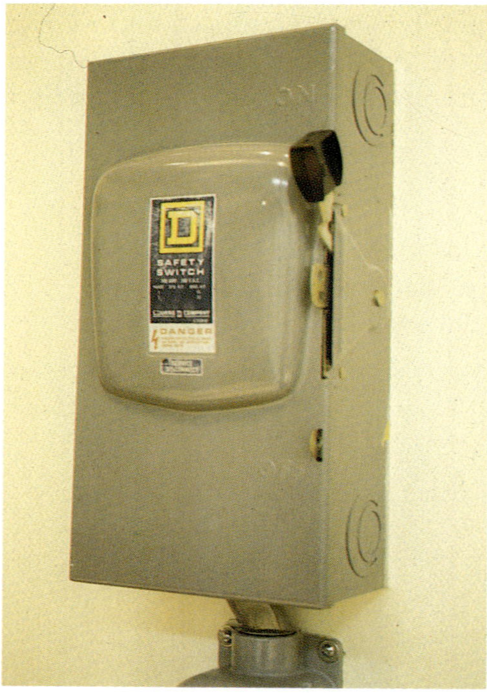

Fig. 34

Insert the fiberoptic connector and secure the connector nut.

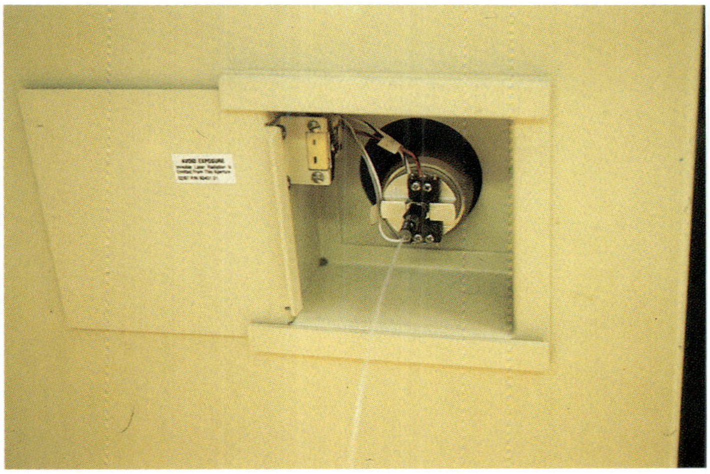

Fig. 35

Release the red emergency button.

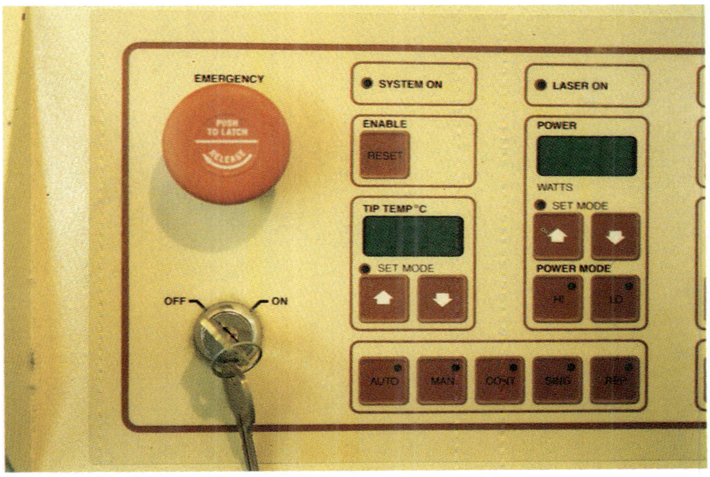

Fig. 36

Insert the key into the keyswitch and turn to the "ON" position by rotating clockwise. Allow four minutes for the machine to warm up. During this phase, make sure that all indicators on the panel show a figure "8".

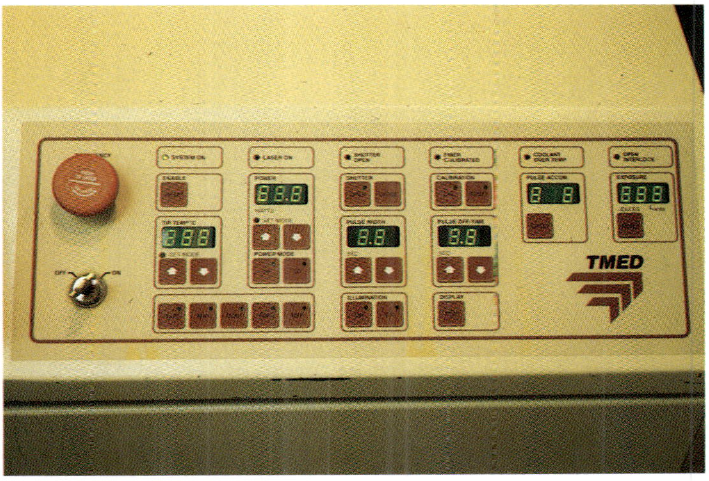

Fig. 37

As soon as the machine is warmed up, all indicators will show a figure "0" and the pre-emission indicator tone will be heard.

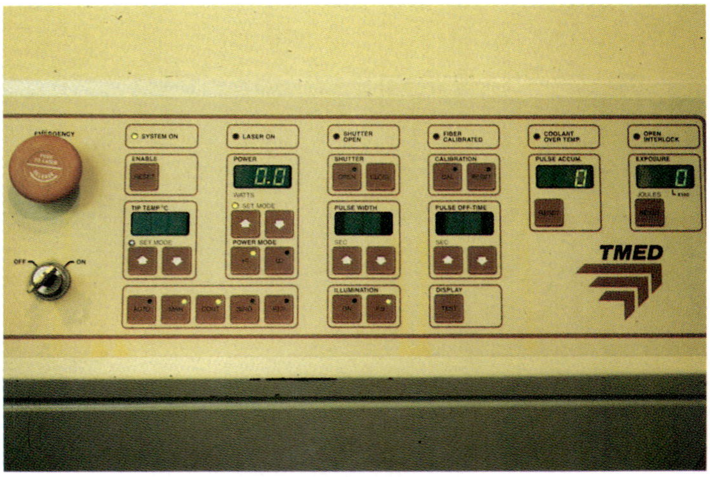

Fig. 38

Push the CONT (continuous mode) switch.

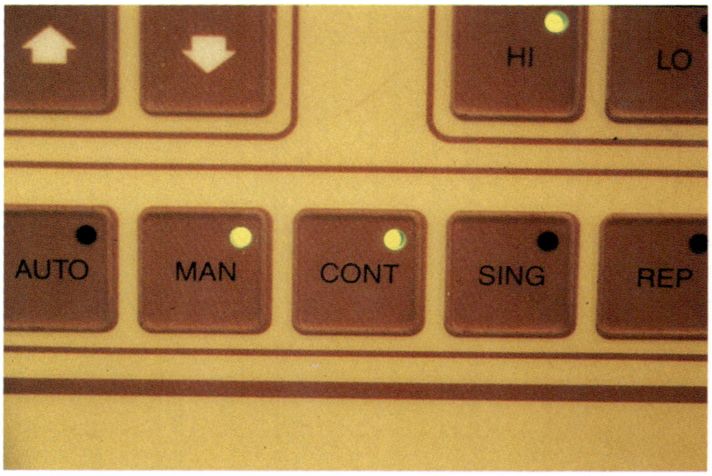

Fig. 39

Then switch to the HI (high) power mode switch.

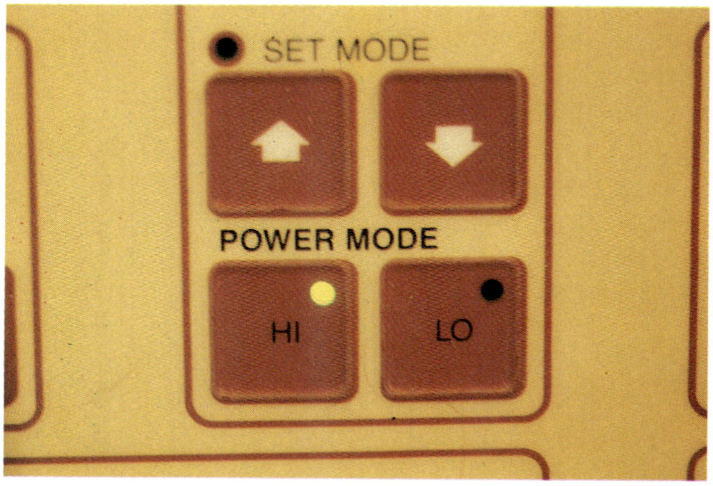

Fig. 40

Select the appropriate power level by using the up or down arrow switch.

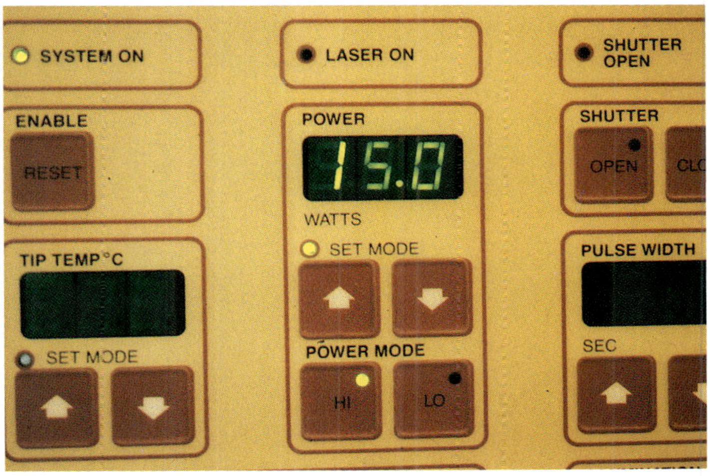

Fig. 41

Appropriate wattages, selected according to the diameters of the distal laser tip, are shown in Table 6. All persons in the room must wear protective eye glasses.

Table 6. Power range of each laser tip.

Laser tip Size (mm)	Appropriate Power Range (watts)
2.5	12-15
3.5	32-34
4.2	32-40
5.0	32-40

After selecting the desired power setting, open the shutter.

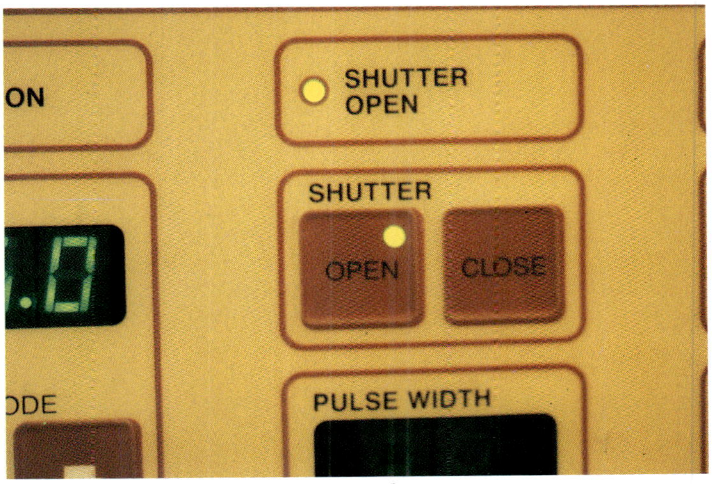

Fig. 42

Depressing the footswitch allows the operator to turn the laser on and easily control lasing time.

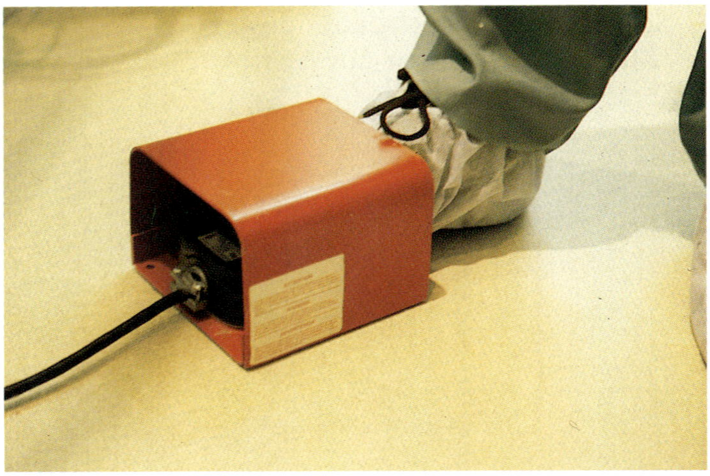

Fig. 43

Before patient application, check the laser function. First, dip the laser tip into a cup filled with saline and depress the footswitch. Activation of the laser tip can be assessed by looking for tiny bubbles all around the tip.

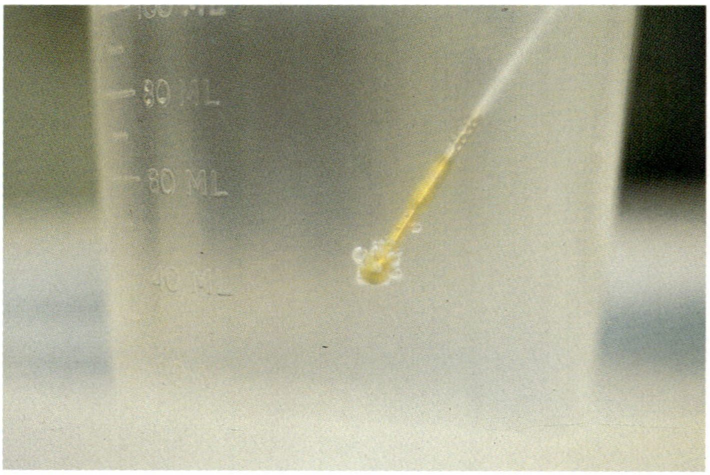

Fig. 44

Usually one laser machine operator, an operating team (two to three doctors, nurses) and a radiology technician with fluoroscope are needed for smooth and successful laser operation.

When the laser machine is not in use during the procedure, the shutter for the laser beam should be turned off for safety.

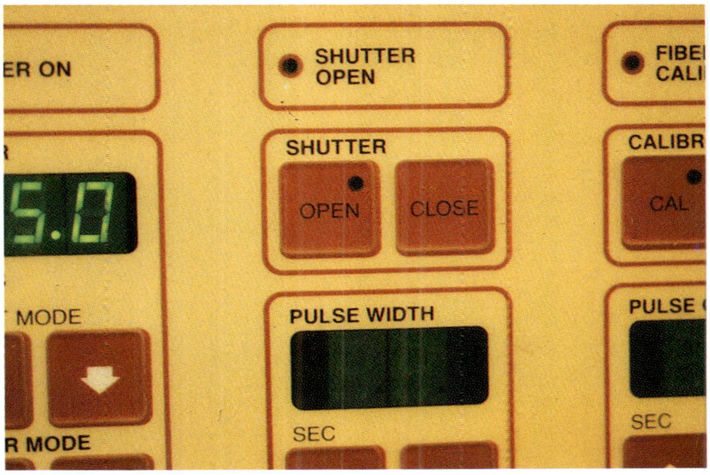

Fig. 45

As soon as the procedure is over, the laser machine should be turned off by turning the laser key counter clockwise and pushing to latch the "release" button.

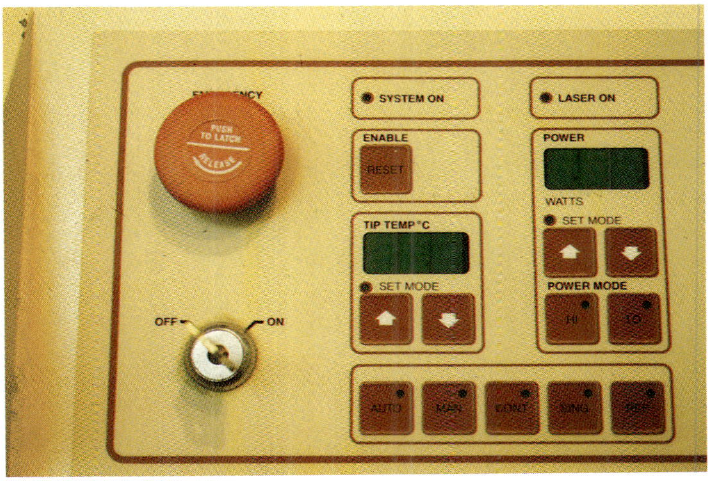

Fig. 46

The power switch should then be turned off and the power source disconnected.

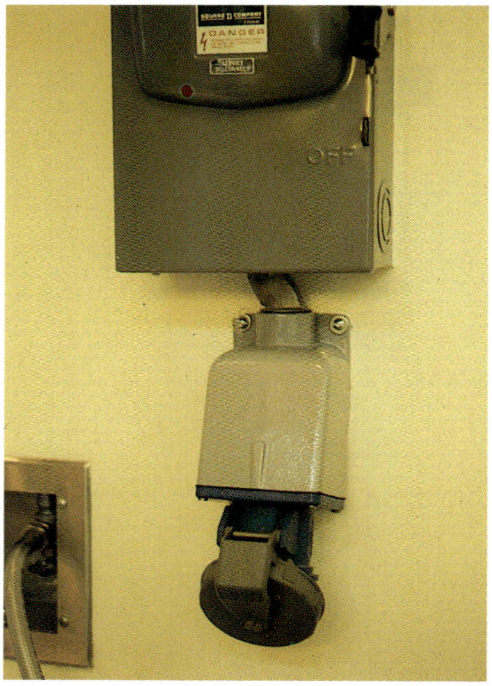

Fig. 47

Circulate water for 20 minutes after use to cool down the machine.

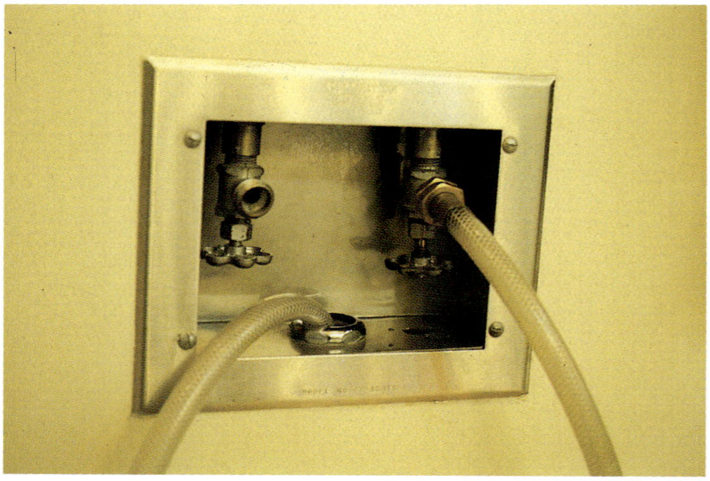

Fig. 48

Chapter 3

THE PERCUTANEOUS APPROACH

Of late, a percutaneous approach[59,62-64] has been used in laser angioplasty and balloon angioplasty for patients having peripheral vascular occlusive disease because of the approach's simplicity and minimum intervention. This approach is preferable in the case of tight stenoses or segmental occlusions of the iliac artery (IA), superficial femoral artery (SFA), and popliteal artery (PA), provided that the common femoral artery (CFA) and the proximal end of the SFA are patent. Being a relatively simple procedure, the percutaneous approach may be tried first, but the surgical approach should be held in reserve in case the percutaneous approach fails. Because of that possibility, all procedures should be performed in the operating suite. Unlike a cutdown procedure, the percutaneous approach can reduce hospitalization time, hospital costs, and morbidity.

Indications

1. Patent CFA or proximal SFA with normal flow.
2. Length of occlusion does not exceed 50% of the SFA.
3. Tight stenosis of common IA, distal SFA, or distal arteries in any length, when a guidewire cannot pass.
4. Non-obese patient.

Procedures

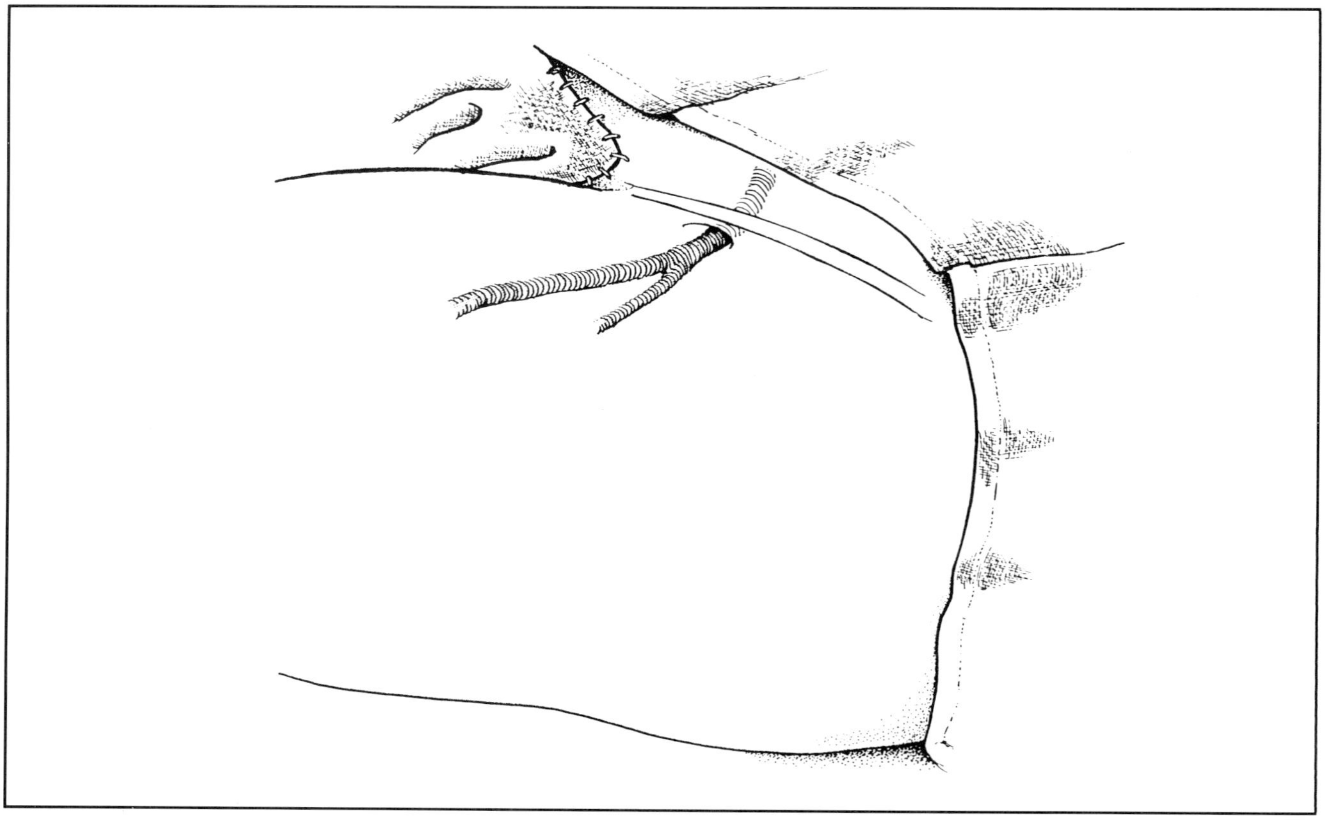

Fig. 49. Under local, epidural or general anesthesia, the lower abdomen, groin and entire lower extremity are prepared and draped.

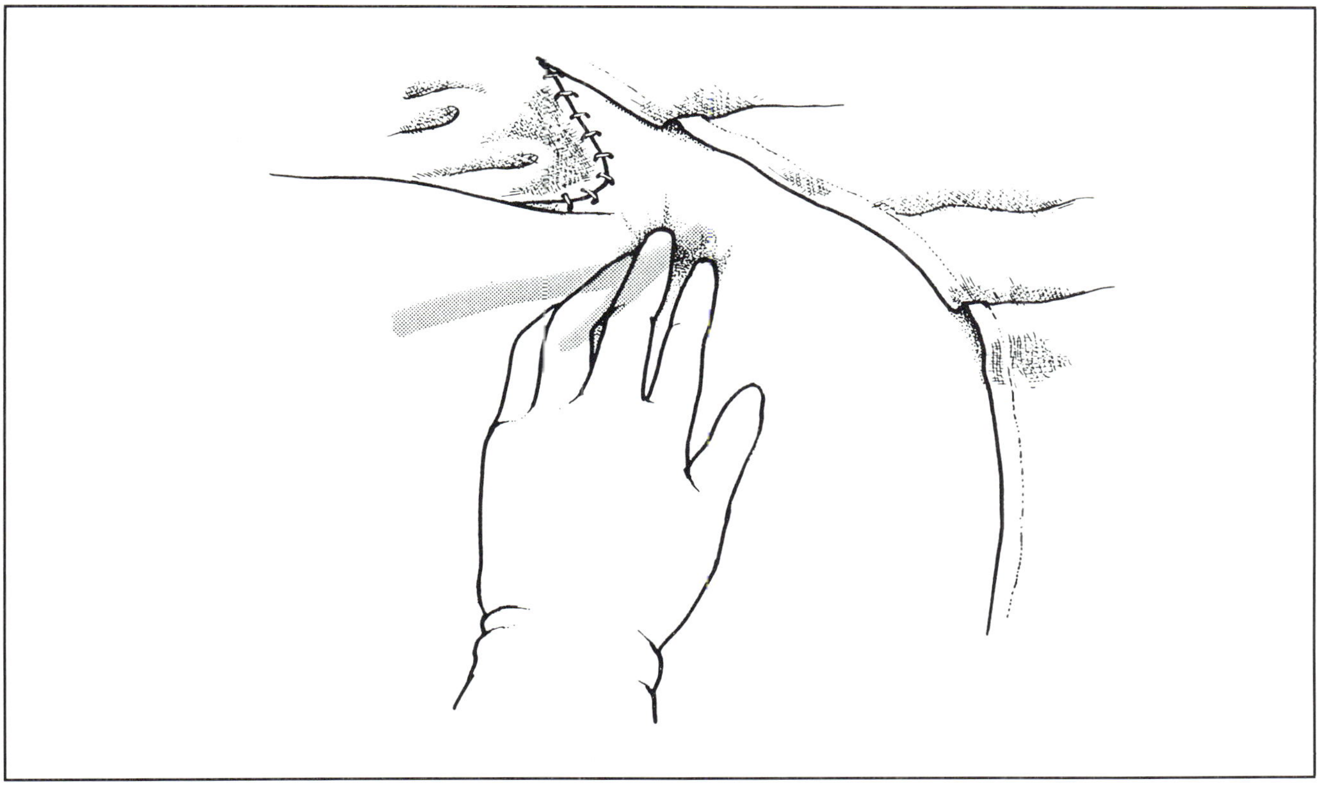

Fig. 50a

The entire foot is covered with a sterile plastic bowel bag. Locations of the audible dorsalis pedis and posterior tibial arteries are clearly marked with durable ink. The CFA is palpated and identified (Fig. 50a and b).

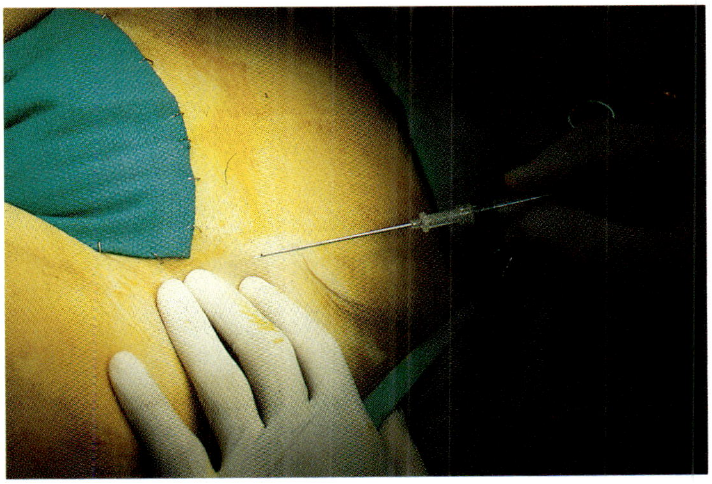

Fig. 50b

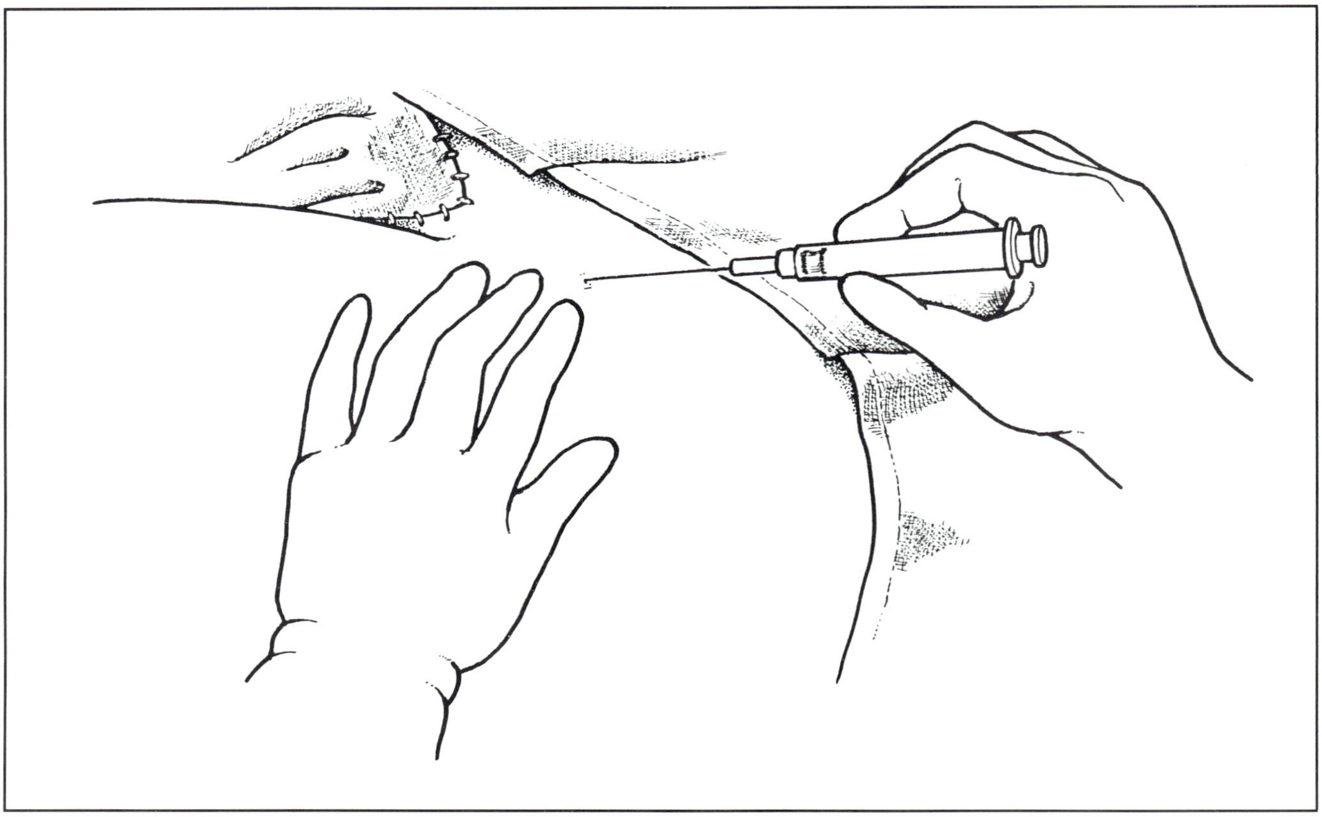

Fig. 51a

The CFA is punctured with an 18 gauge Cournand needle (Fig. 51a and b).

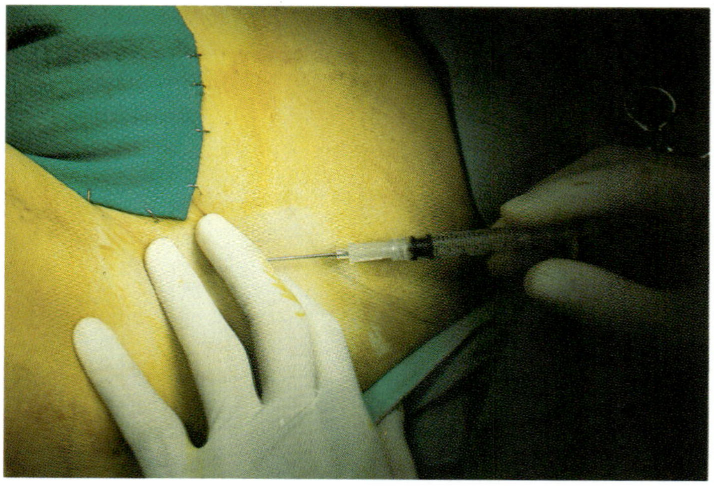

Fig. 51b

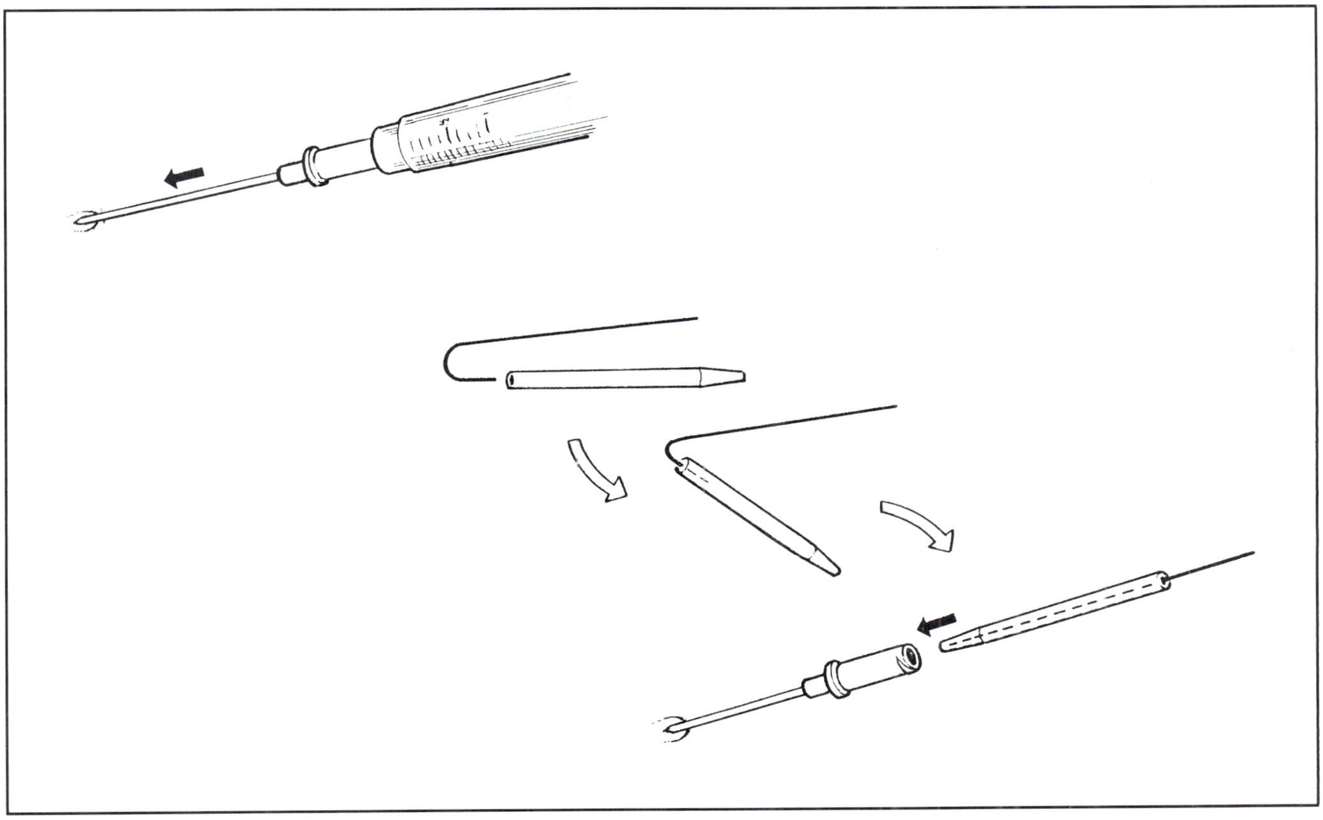

Fig. 52a

A J-guidewire (0.89-mm diameter, 45-cm long) is introduced through the needle (Fig. 52a and b).

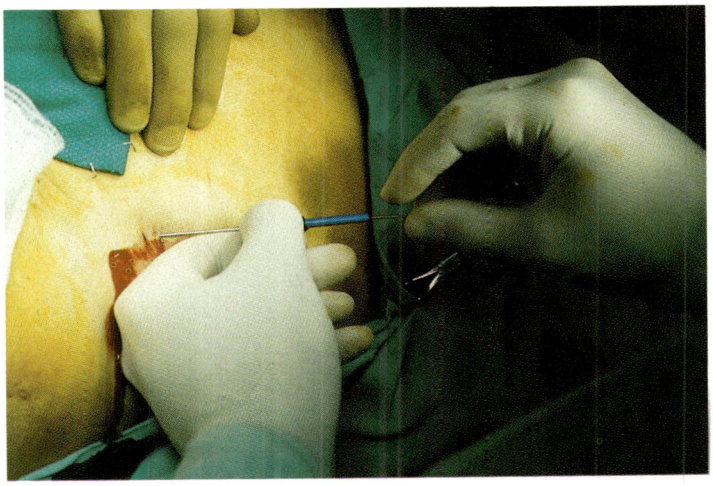

Fig. 52b

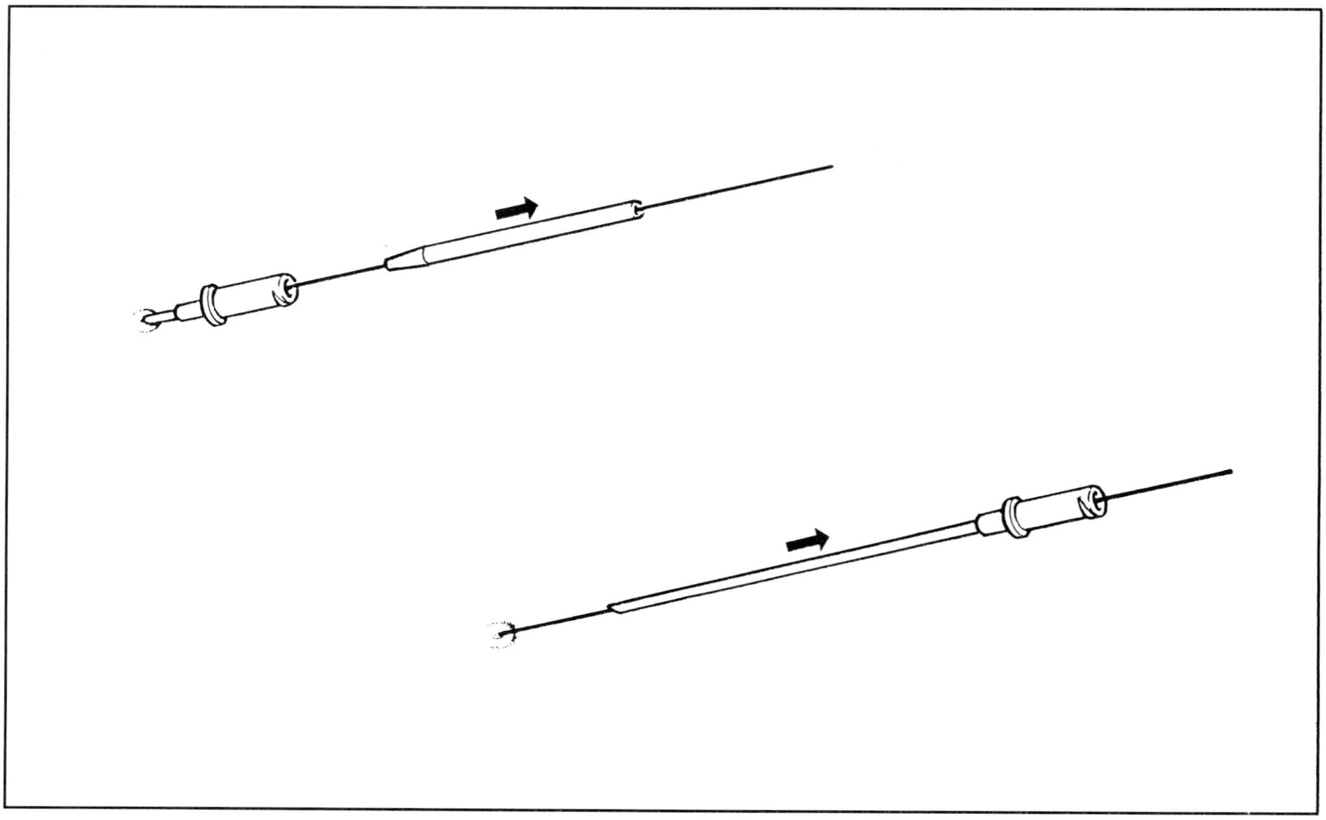

Fig. 53. The needle is removed leaving the guidewire in the arterial lumen.

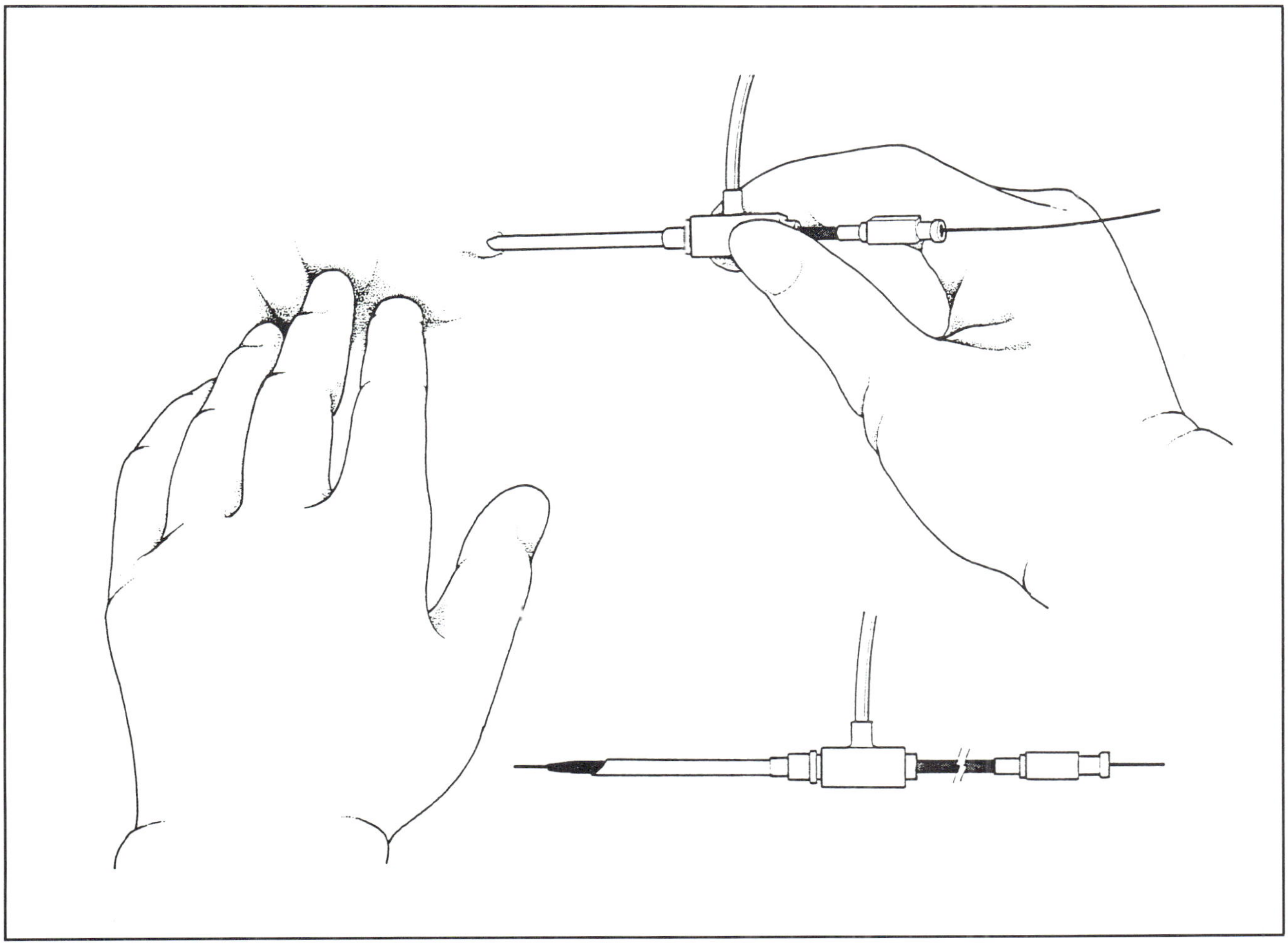

Fig. 54a

The French introducer sheath with black introducer is slipped over the J-guidewire and advanced until the distal end of the French introducer reaches the arterial lumen (Fig. 54a and b).

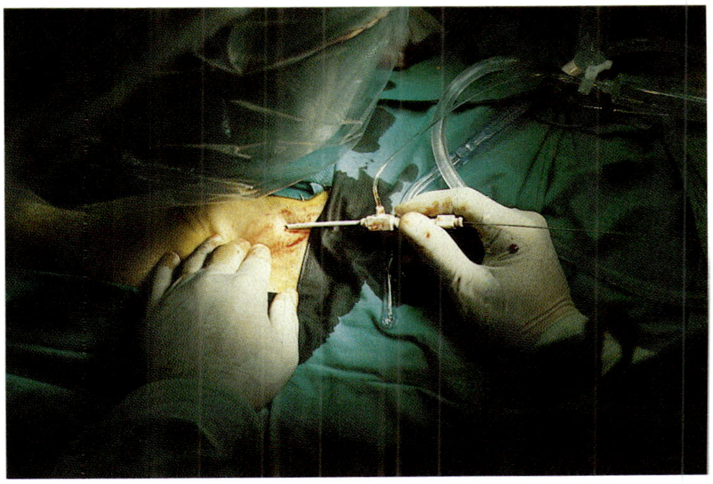

Fig. 54b

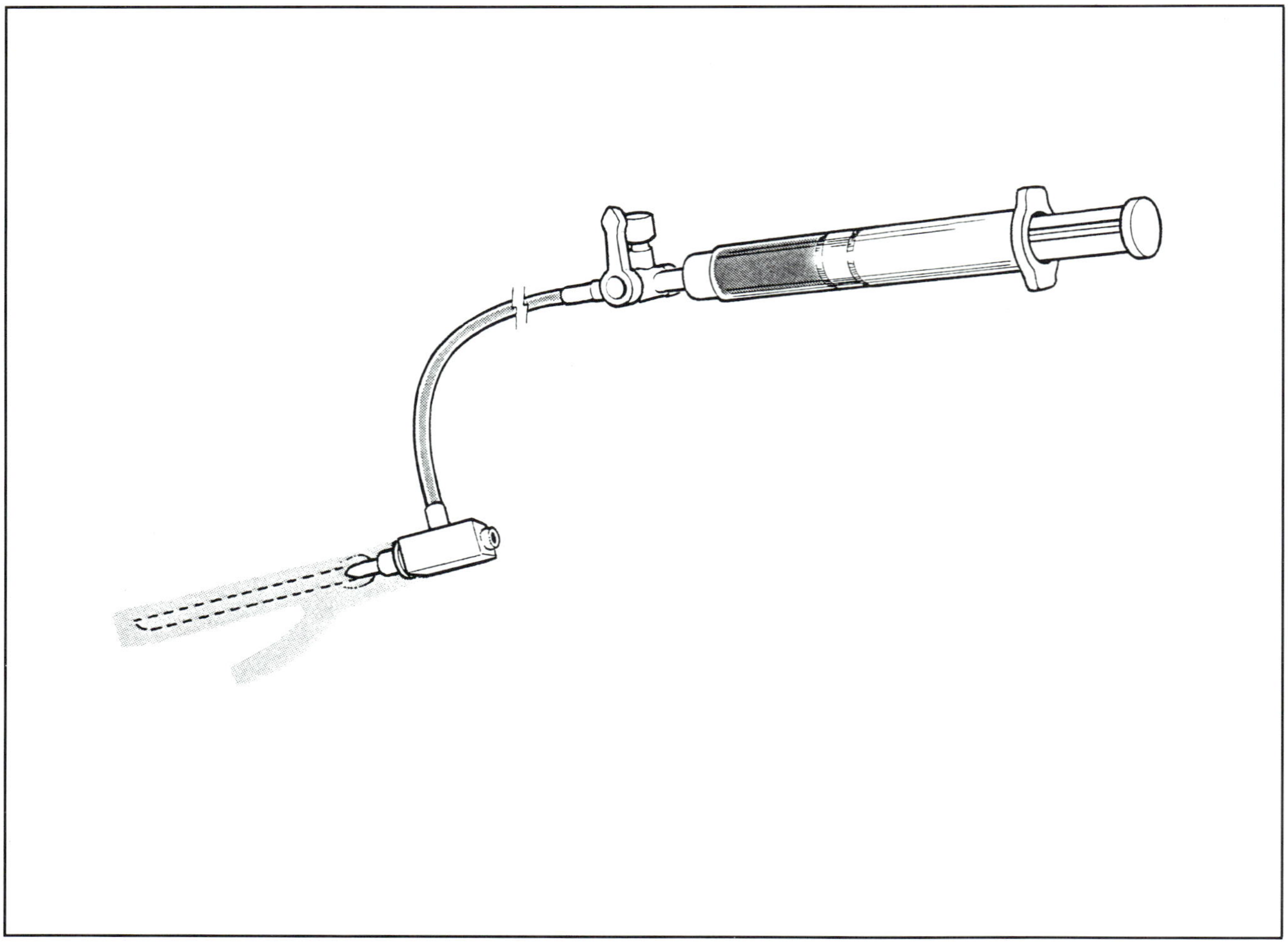

Fig. 55a

This location is confirmed by backflow of blood into the side port tube (Fig. 55a and b).

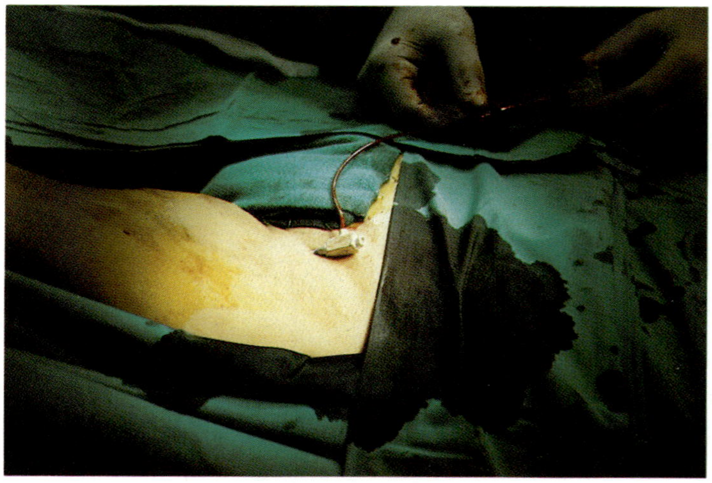

Fig. 55b

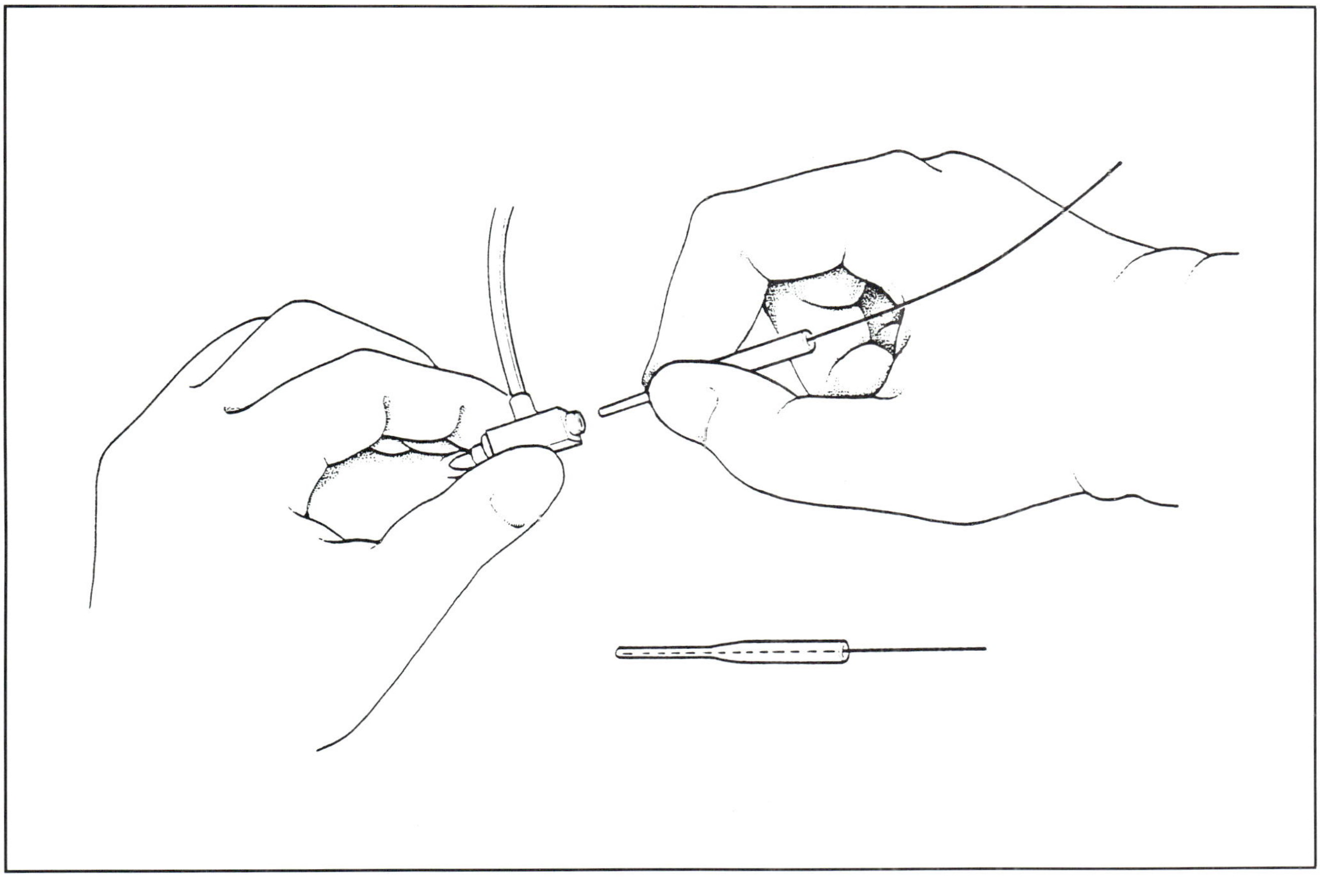

Fig. 56a

After removing the J-guidewire, a hydrophilic guidewire (0.89-mm diameter, 150-cm long) is introduced into the arterial lumen through the sheath (Fig. 56a and b).

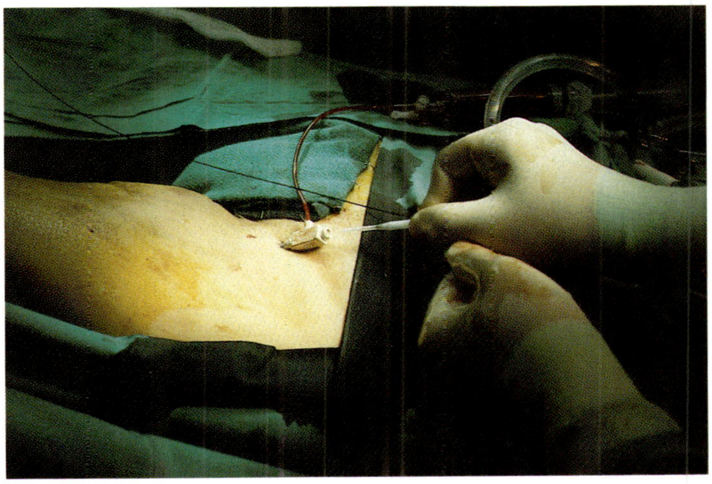

Fig. 56b

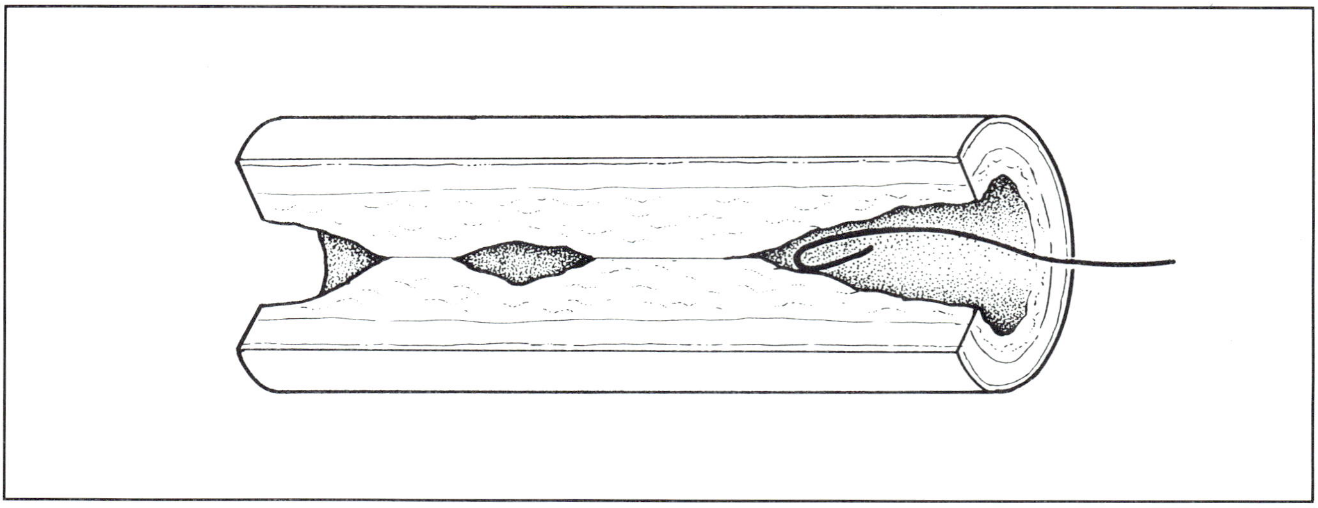

Fig. 57a

The guidewire is negotiated through the occlusive lesion under fluoroscopy (Fig. 57a and b).

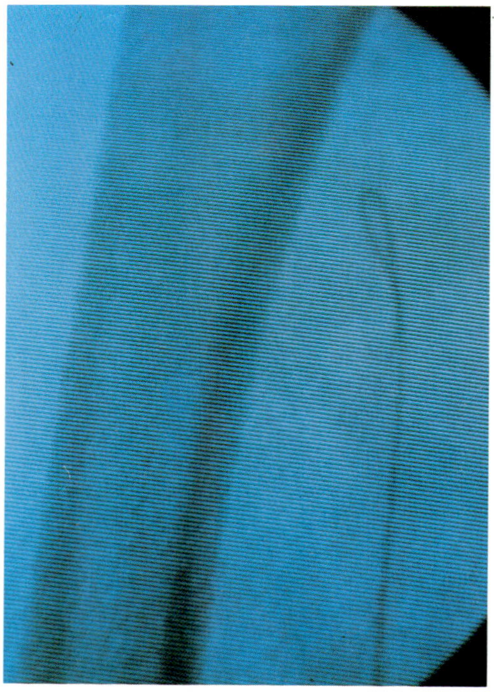

Fig. 57b

When the guidewire cannot pass through the lesion, laser recanalization is performed. Before turning on the laser machine, make sure that EVERYONE in the operative suite is wearing protective glasses and all windows in the operating room are covered. Then the laser machine may be activated as described in chapter I or II.

Before using the laser probe on the patient, test for probe activation by dipping the probe into saline and observing bubble formation around the activated laser tip.

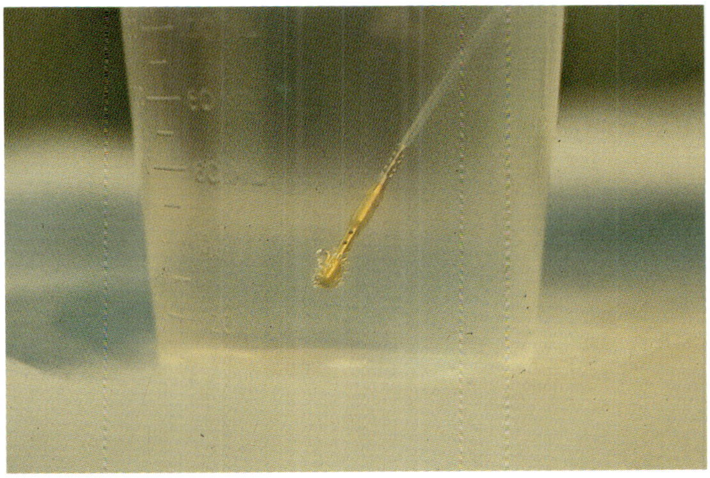

Fig. 58

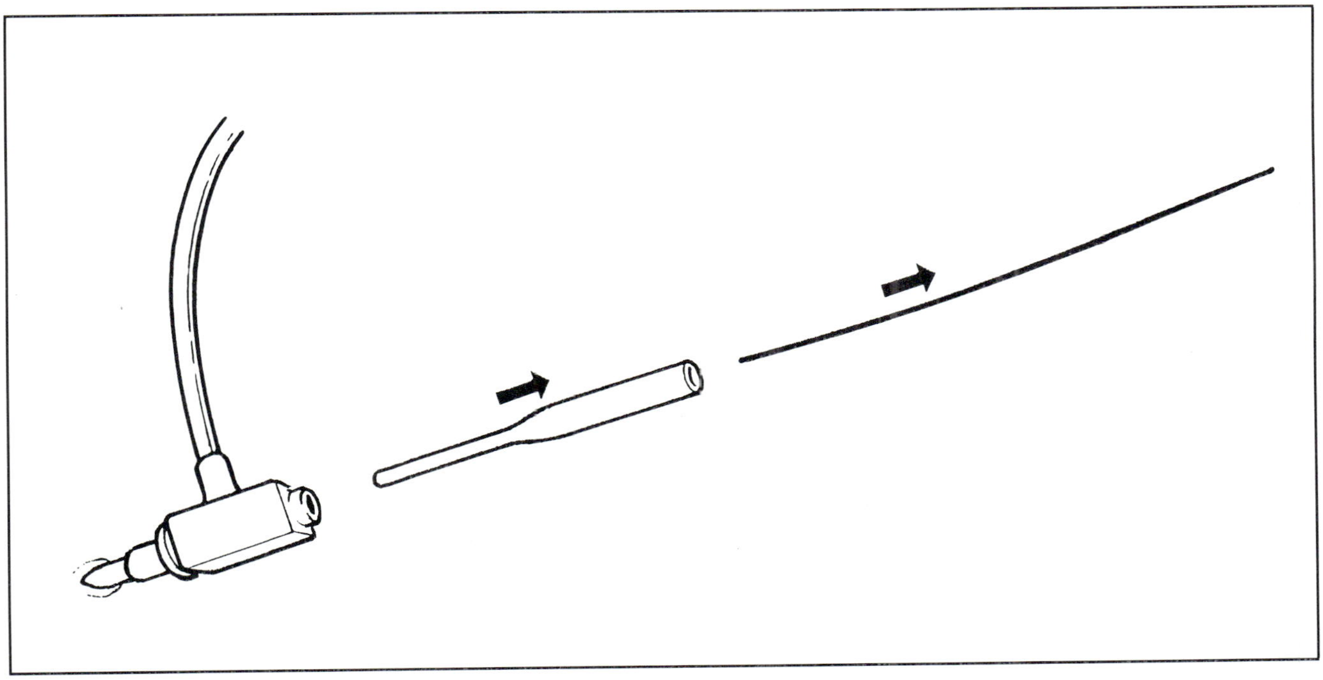

Fig. 59. The hydrophilic guidewire is pulled out.

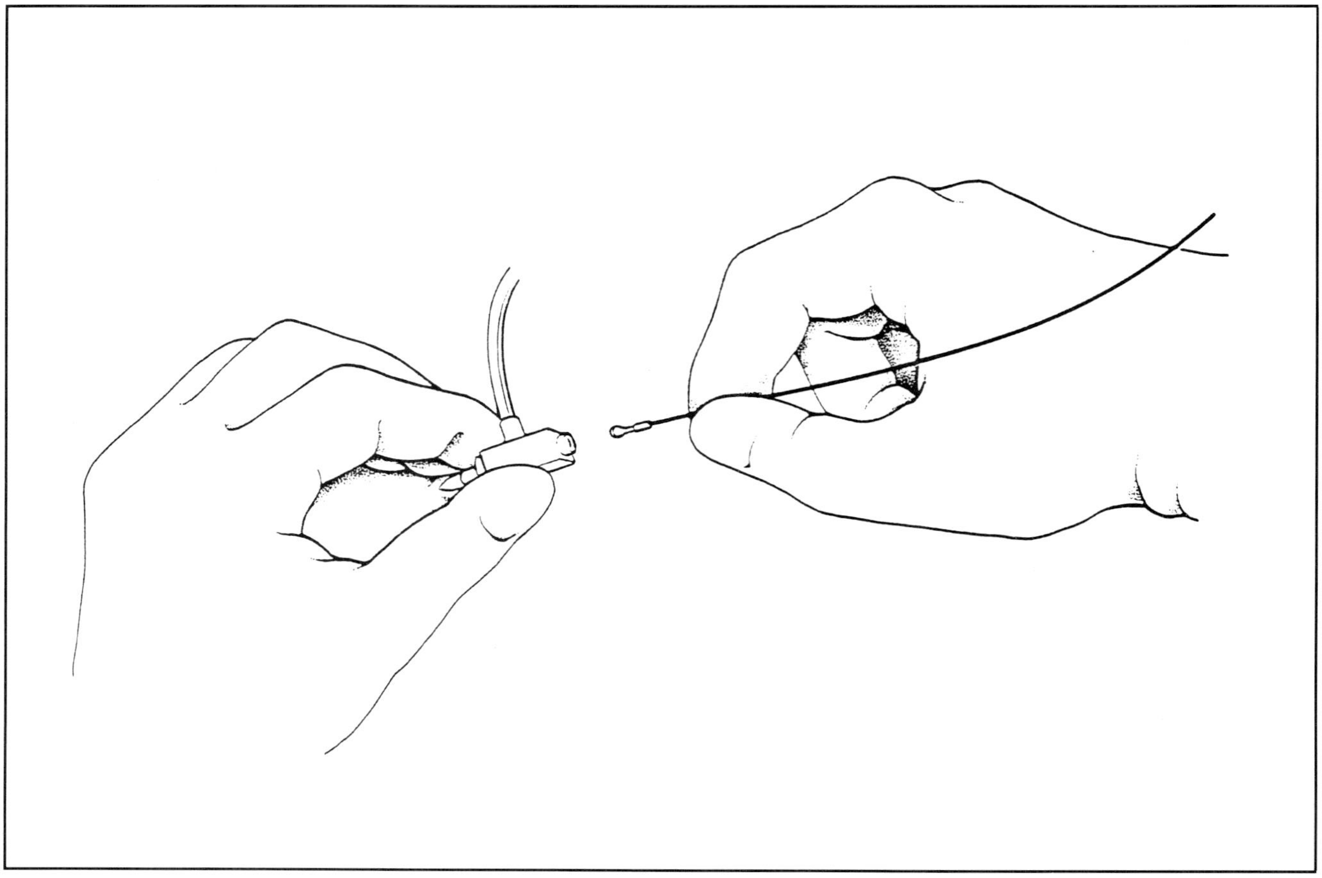

Fig. 60. The 2.5-mm laser probe is inserted through the introducer sheath.

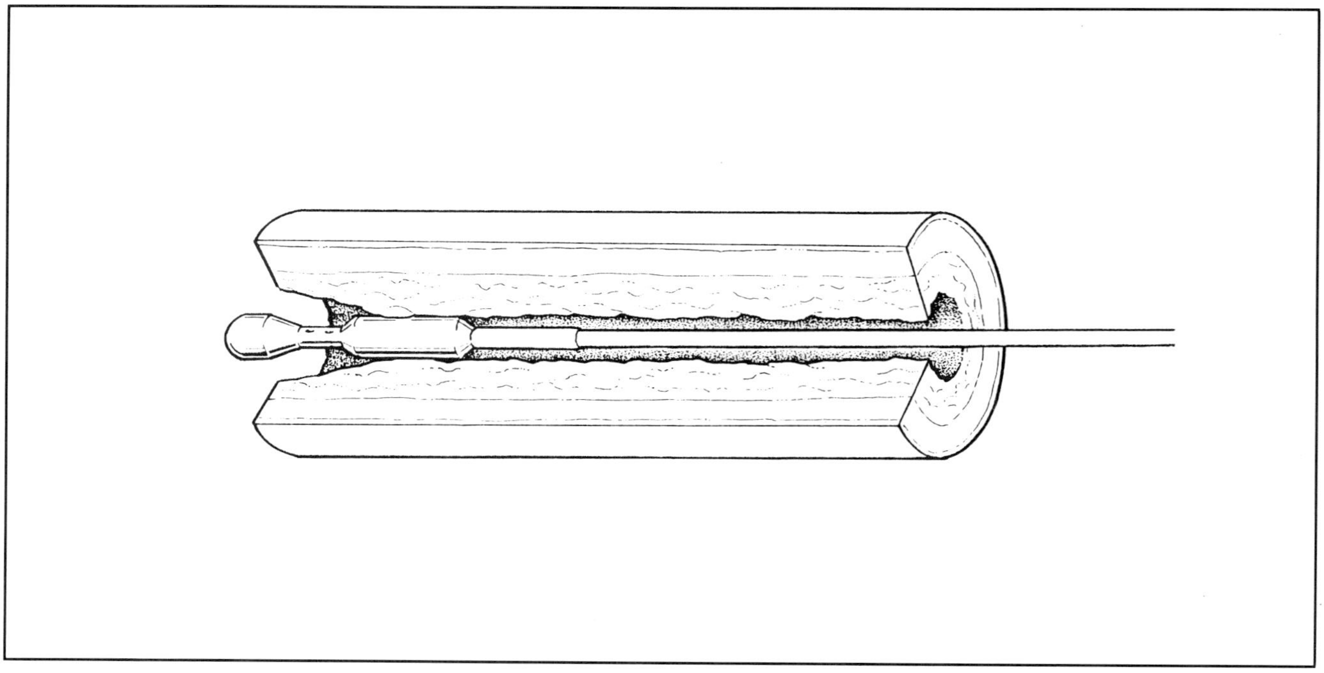

Fig. 61a

The probe is moved in a back-and-forth motion under fluoroscopy (Fig. 61a and b).

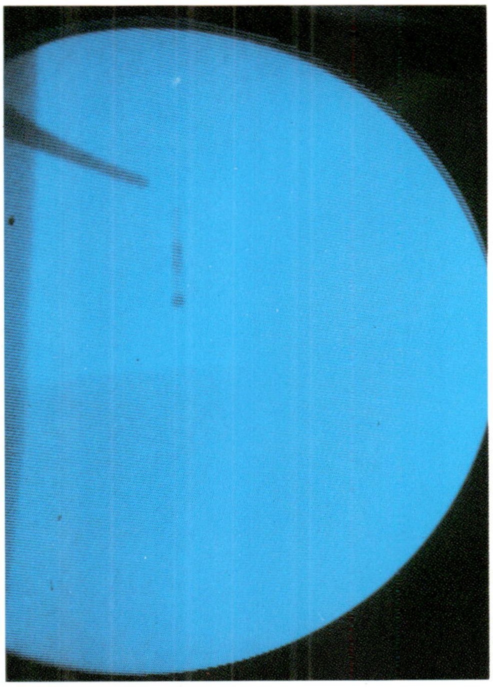

Fig. 61b

When advancing the laser probe, contrast medium is periodically injected to confirm the creation of a new channel or detect complications such as perforation while using fluoroscopy.

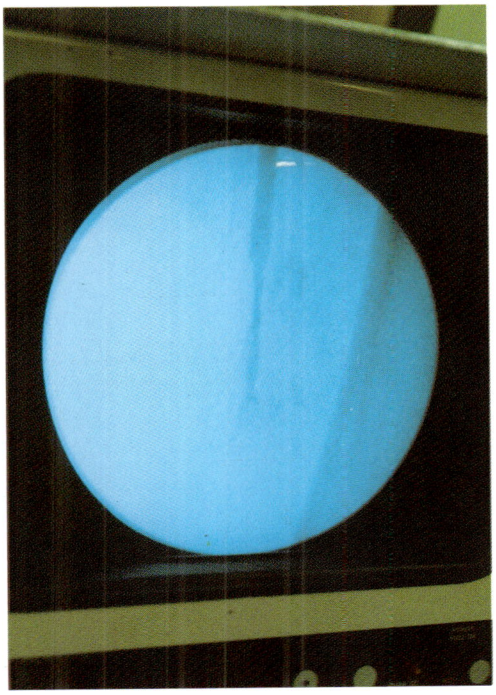

Fig. 62

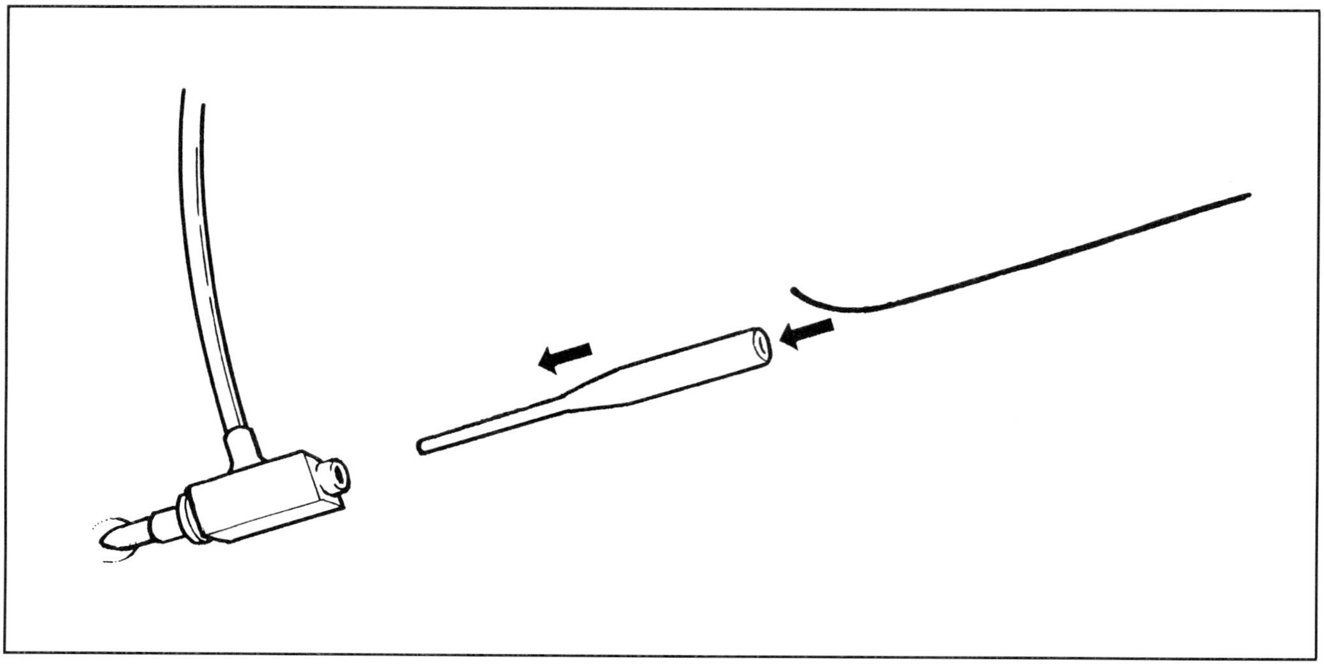

Fig. 63. After the laser recanalization, a hydrophilic guidewire is passed through to insure a new channel through the lesion.

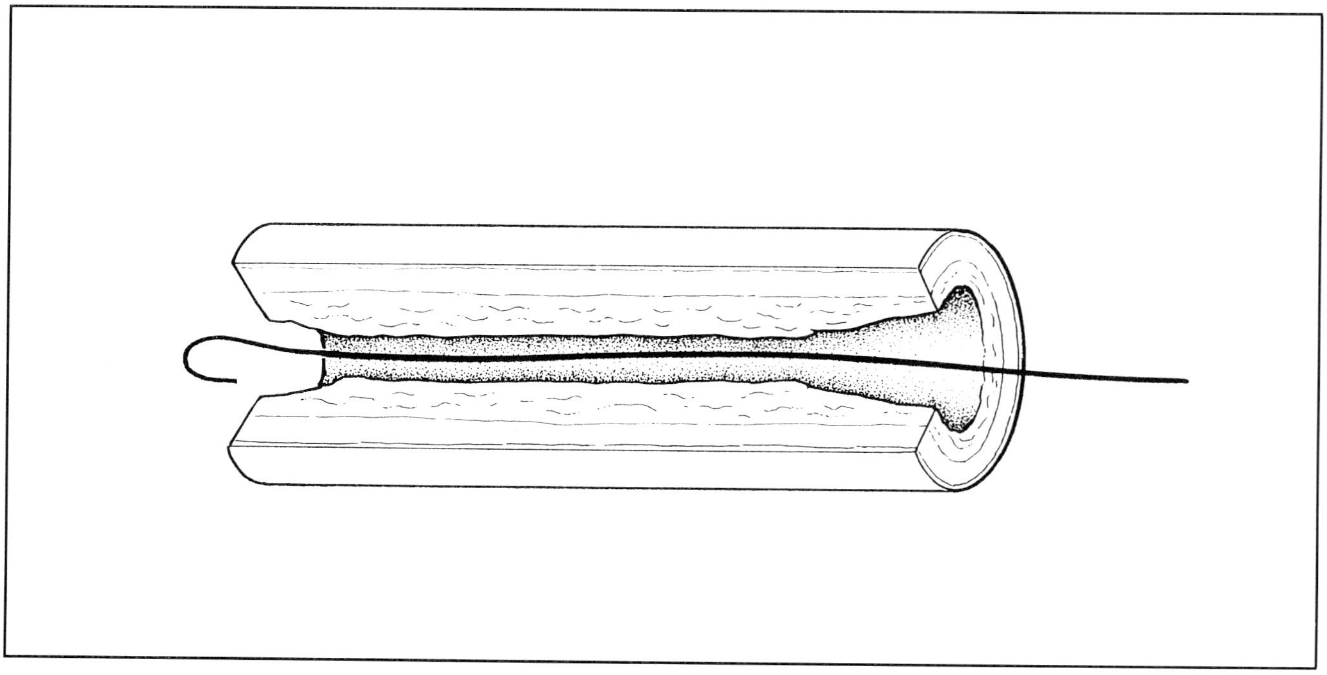

Fig. 64a

The guidewire is then advanced distally through the newly created channel to facilitate procedures such as balloon dilatation (see chapter V) (Fig. 64a and b).

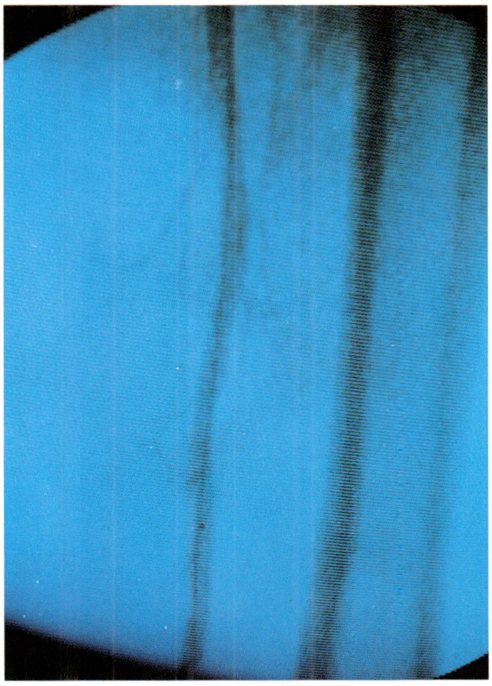

Fig. 64b

Complications of the Approach

1. Infection at puncture site
2. Hematoma
3. Damage to adjacent structures such as the femoral nerve or femoral vein by the needle
4. Pseudoaneurysm
5. Extravasation of the contrast medium with edema of the lower extremity

Chapter 4

SURGICAL APPROACH (CUT-DOWN PROCEDURE)

The percutaneous approach, being simpler than the surgical approach, should be considered in all cases, although it may not be deemed feasible in all cases. A surgical cut-down may provide ready access if the percutaneous approach fails; however, if this procedure also fails or causes complications, a bypass procedure is then necessary. The entire procedure, therefore, should be undertaken in an operating suite with proper advance preparation.

In the case of stenosis of the CFA or proximal SFA, the percutaneous approach is virtually impossible because insertion of the needle into the arterial lumen will not only be difficult to place exactly, but will increase the risk of dissection of the calcified intimal layer. In a markedly obese patient, identification, fixation and puncture of the CFA is difficult even with the aid of a Doppler. In the case of extended occlusions such as SFA and distal arteries occlusions, the surgical approach is preferable. The surgical approach is more invasive, but it is safer and more reliable in placing the guidewire precisely, with direct vision into the arterial lumen.

Indications for Surgical Approach

1. Markedly obese patients
2. Occlusion, stenosis, or both, of the CFA or proximal end of the SFA
3. Long occlusion more than 2/3 length of the SFA
4. Absence of distal runoff along with SFA occlusion

Procedures

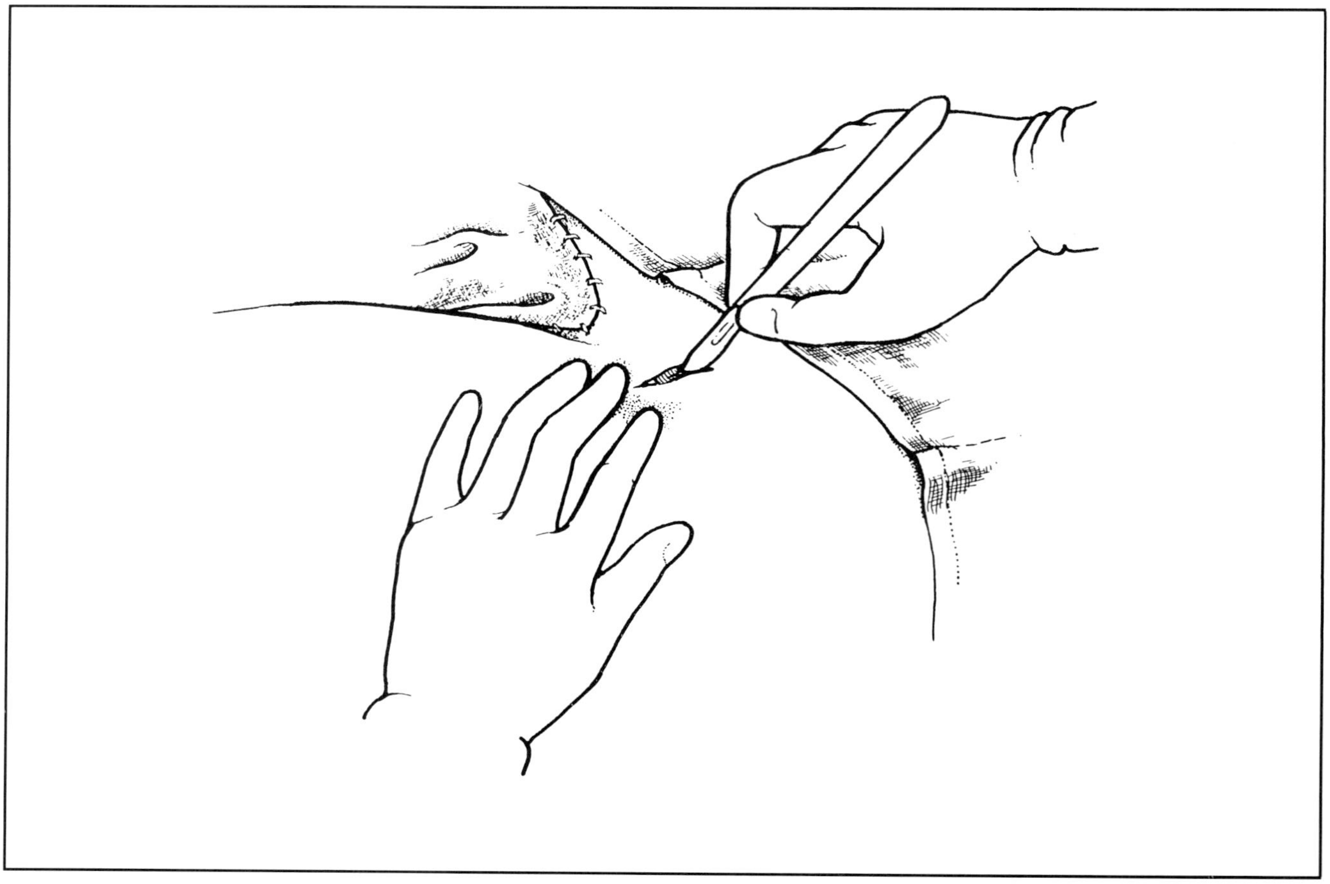

Fig. 65. A longitudinal incision is made at the left groin after sterilization and draping.

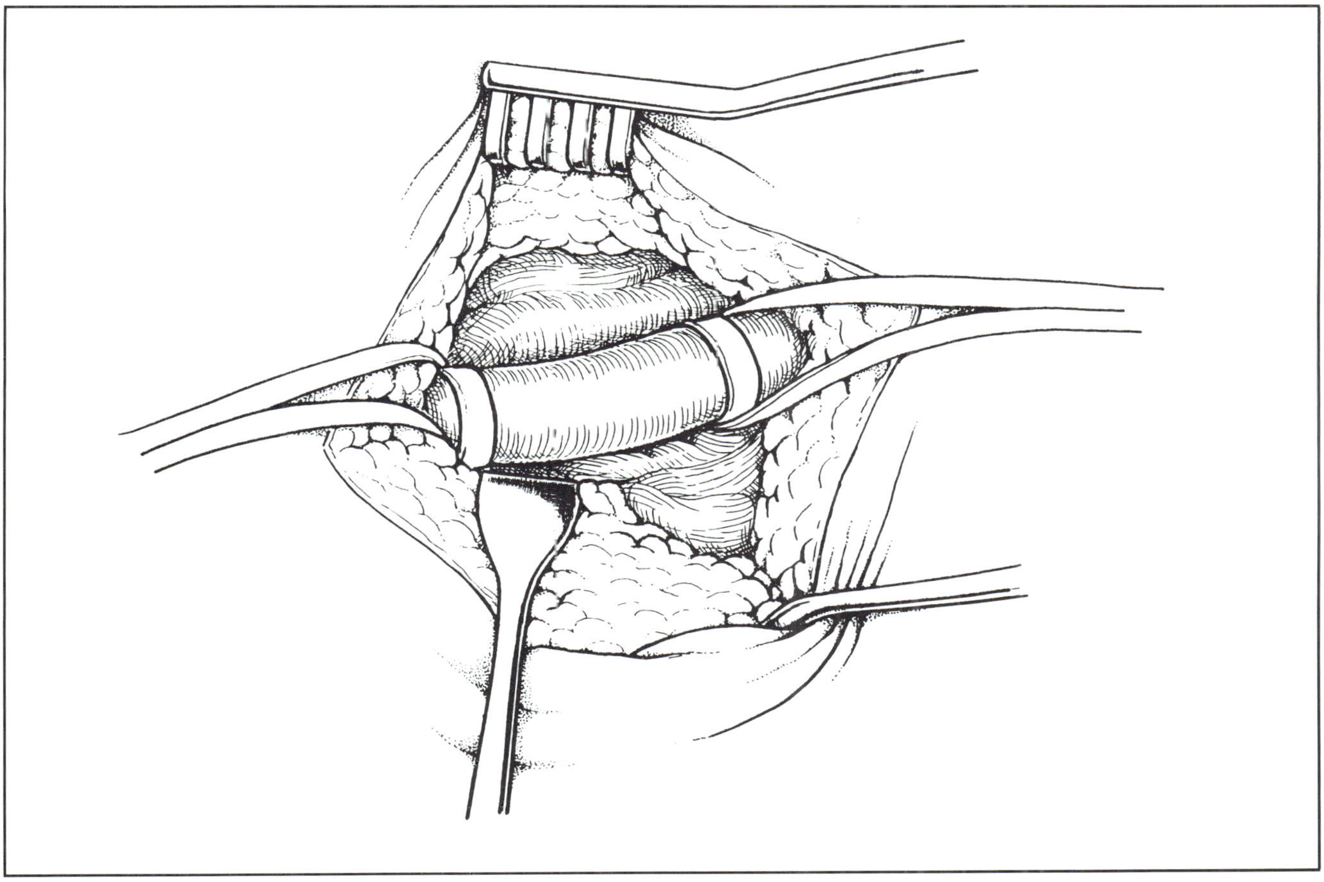

Fig. 66a

The CFA is then identified and isolated. Vessel loops are used at the proximal and distal ends of the exposed artery (Fig. 66a and b).

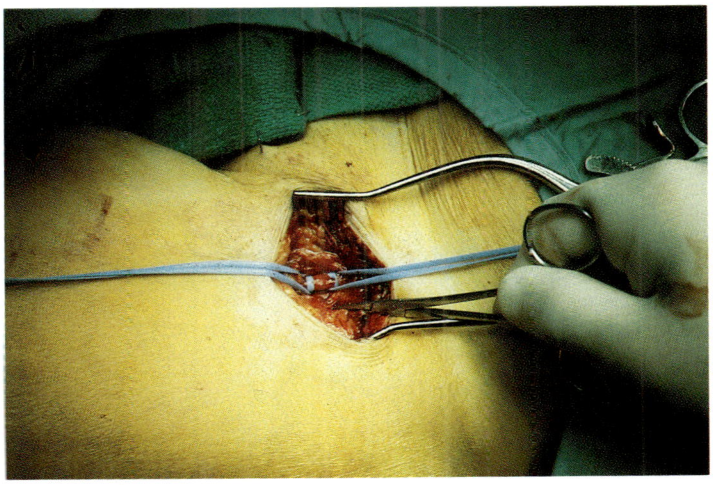

Fig. 66b

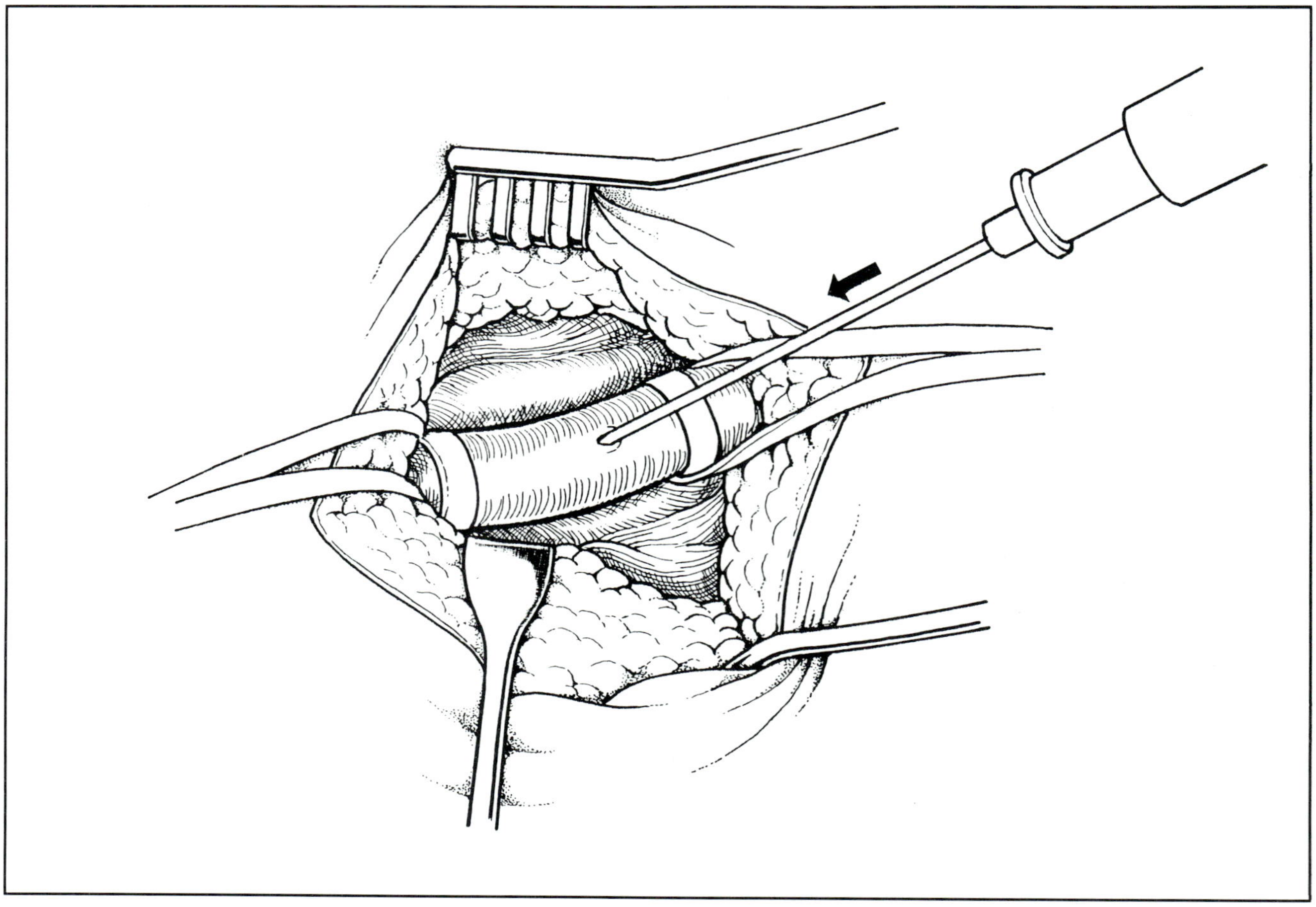

Fig. 67a

Thc CFA is punctured using an 18-gauge Cournand needle (Fig. 67a and b).

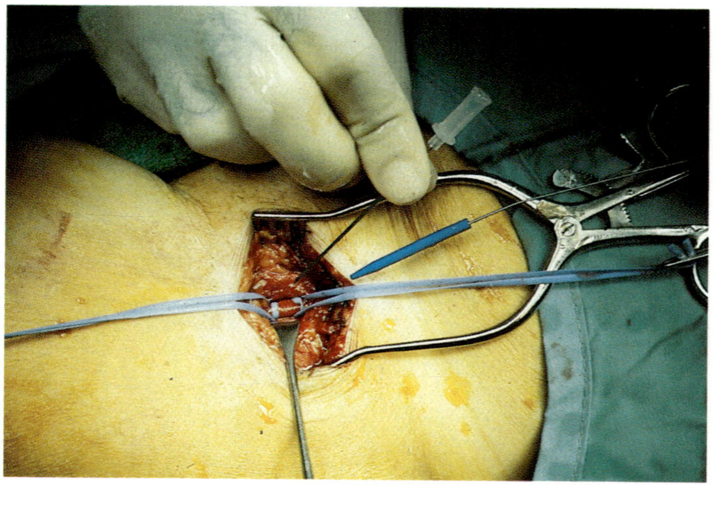

Fig. 67b

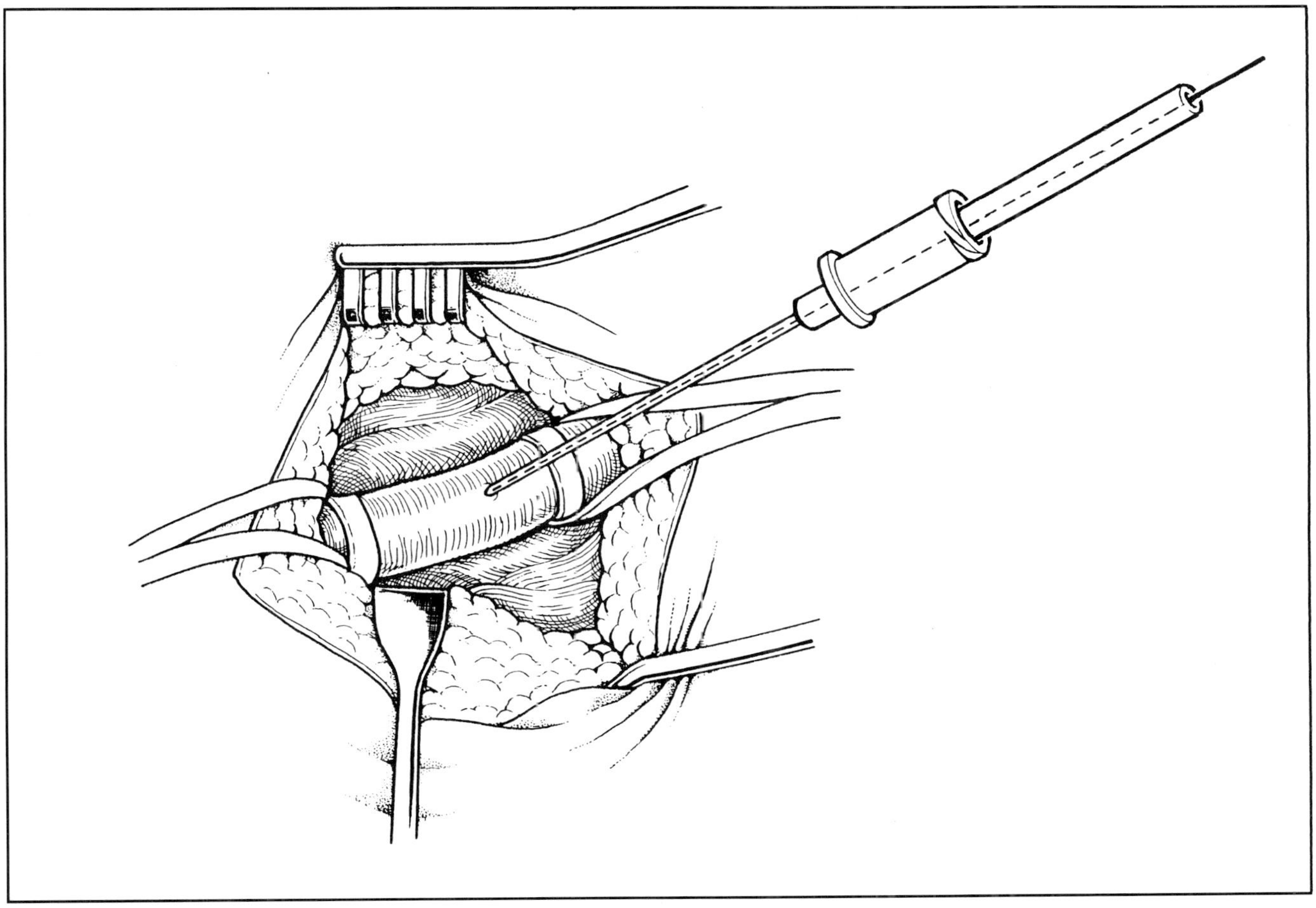

Fig. 68. A J-guidewire (0.89-mm diameter and 45-cm long) is introduced into the arterial lumen through the needle.

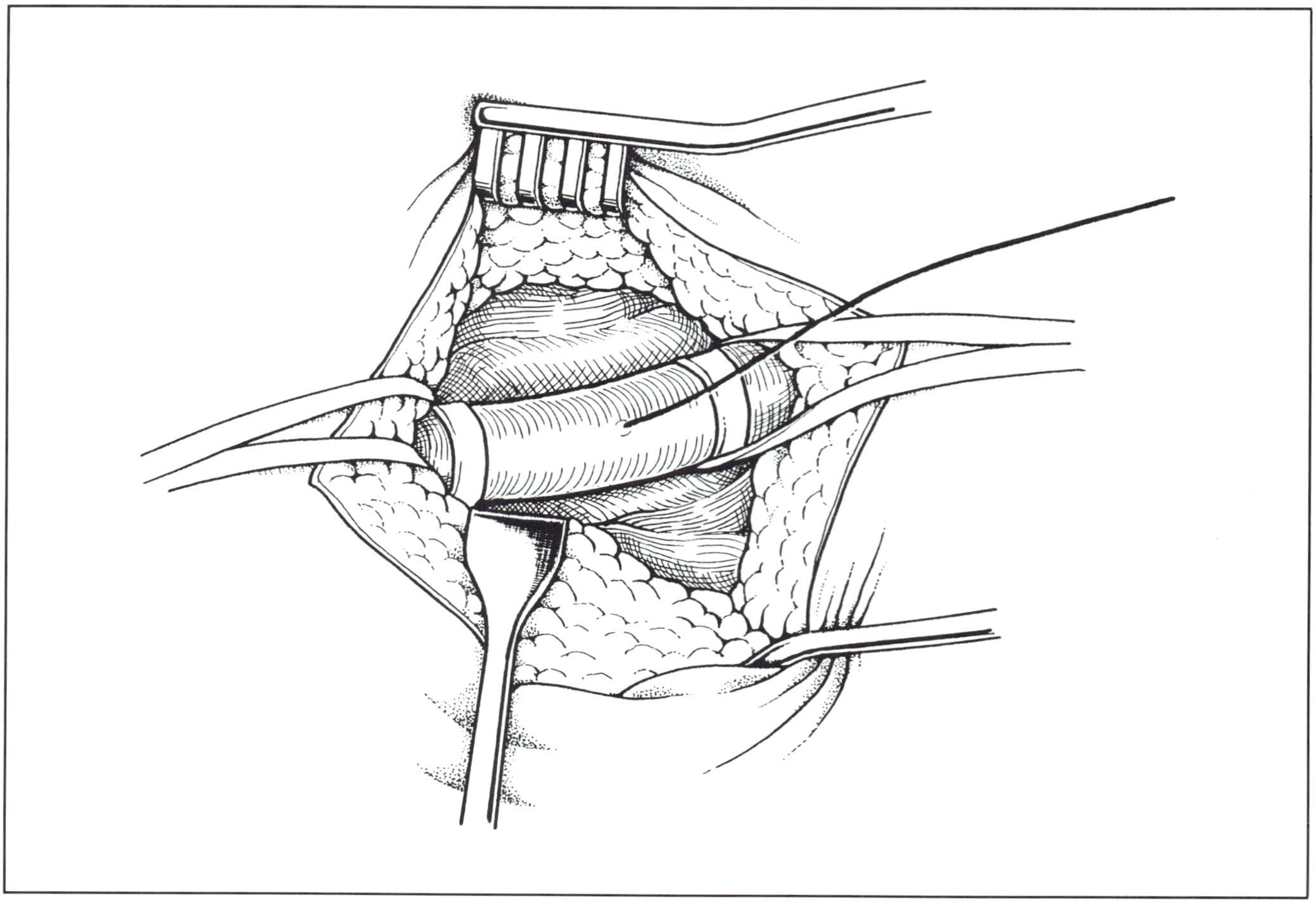

Fig. 69a

The needle is removed, leaving the guidewire in the arterial lumen (Fig. 69a and b).

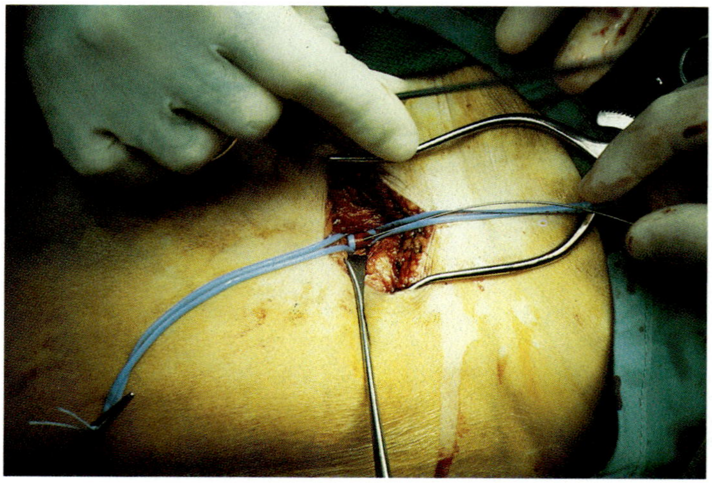

Fig. 69b

The French introducer sheath is cut according to the patency length of the proximal SFA.

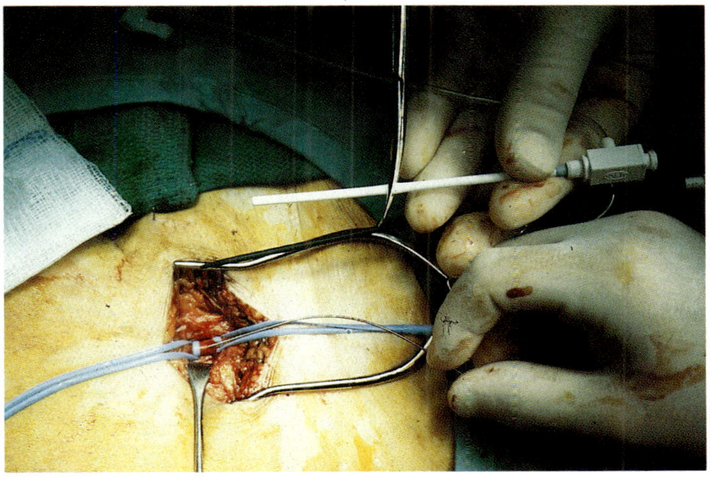

Fig. 70

The sheath is then attached to the introducer...

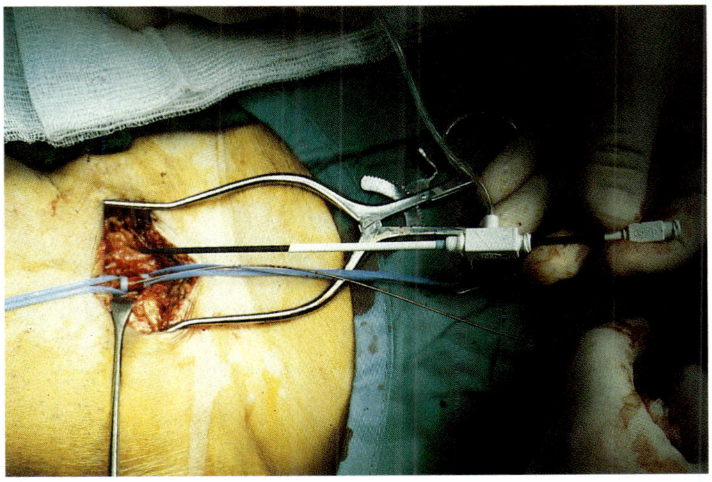

Fig. 71

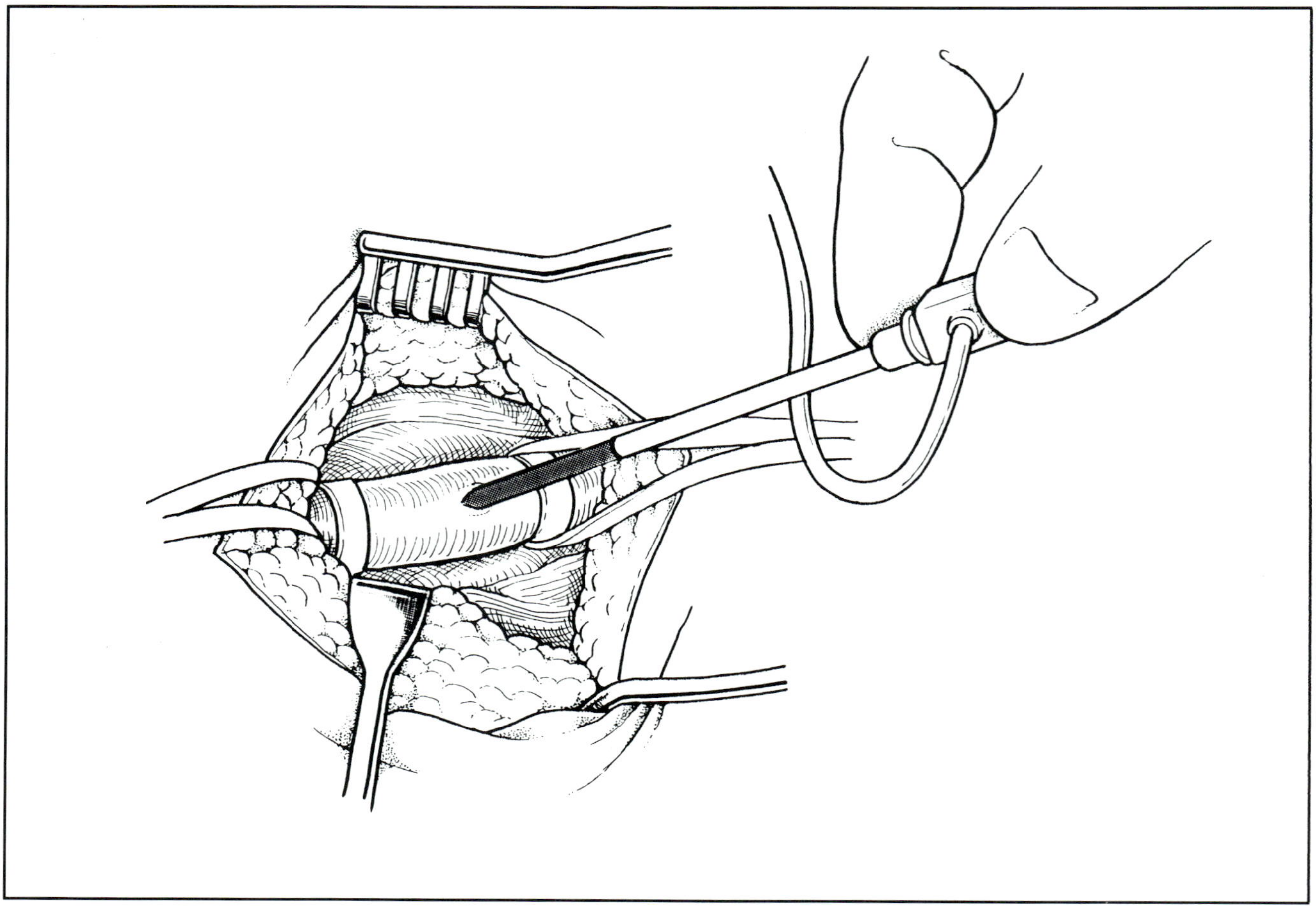

Fig. 72a

and slipped over the guide wire into the common femoral artery and advanced further into the SFA lumen (Fig. 72a and b).

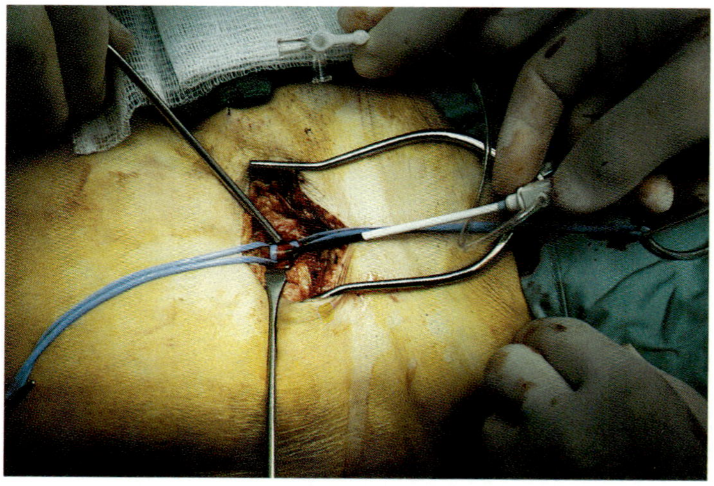

Fig. 72b

Intra-arterial positioning of the sheath is confirmed by back-flow of blood into the side port.

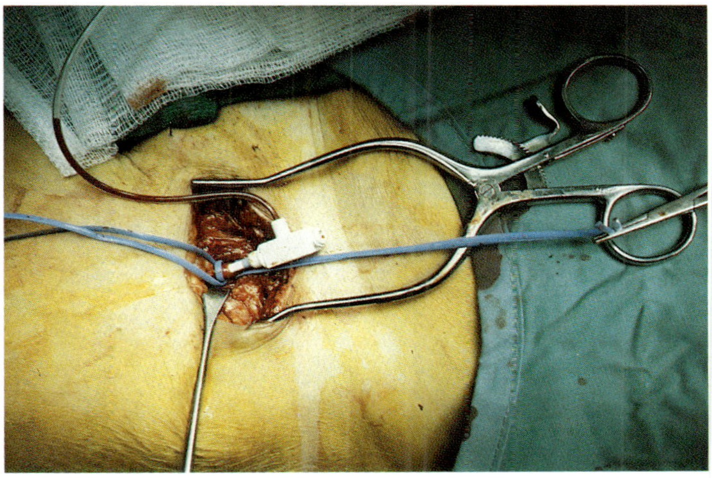

Fig. 73

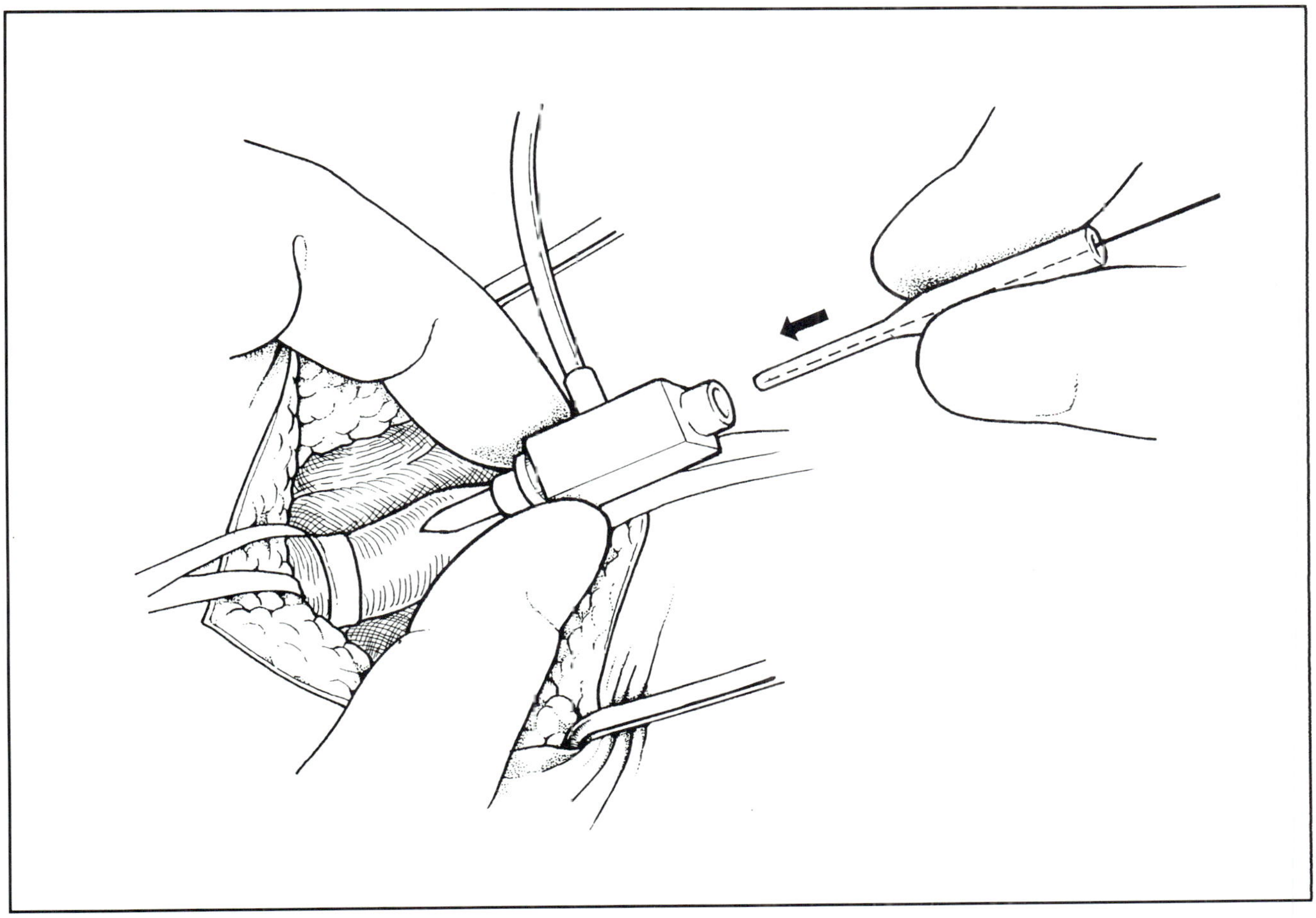

Fig. 74a

After removal of the J guidewire, a hydrophilic guide wire (0.89-mm diameter, 150-cm long) is introduced through the sheath (Fig. 74a and b).

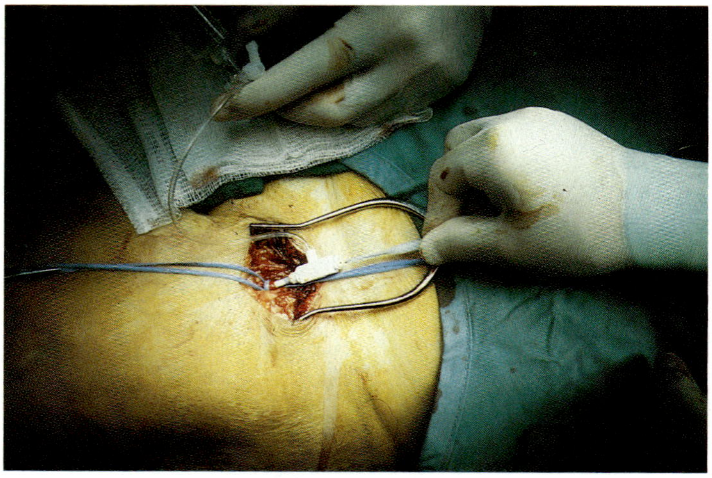

Fig. 74b

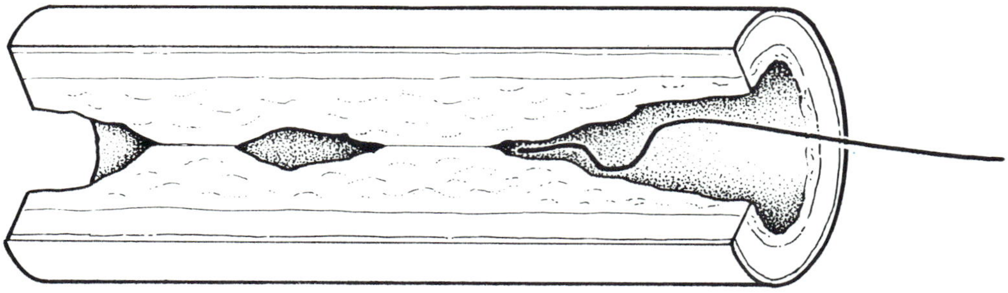

Fig. 75. The guidewire is negotiated through the occlusive lesion under fluoroscopy. If this procedure fails, then laser recanalization is considered.

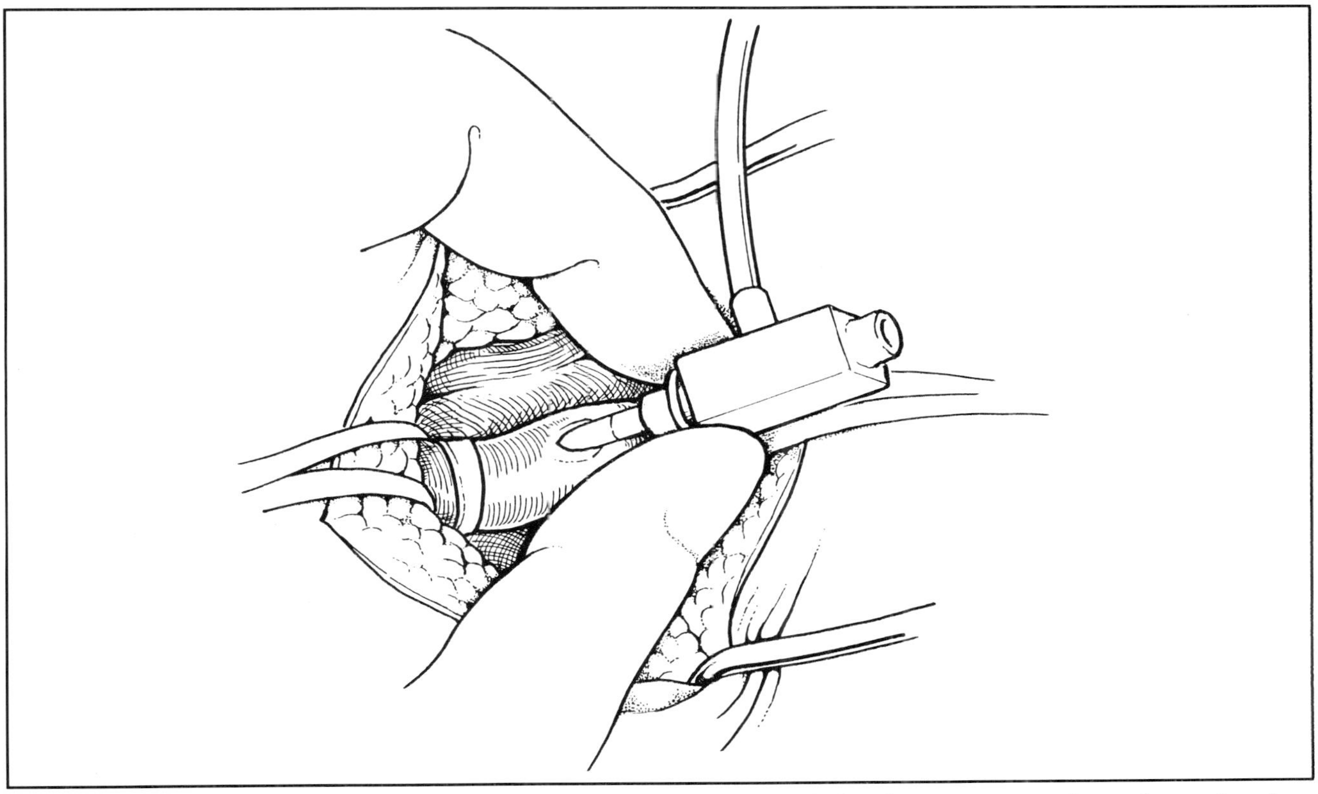

Fig. 76. The hydrophilic guidewire is then removed, and the laser system is activated using all precautions mentioned in Chapter II.

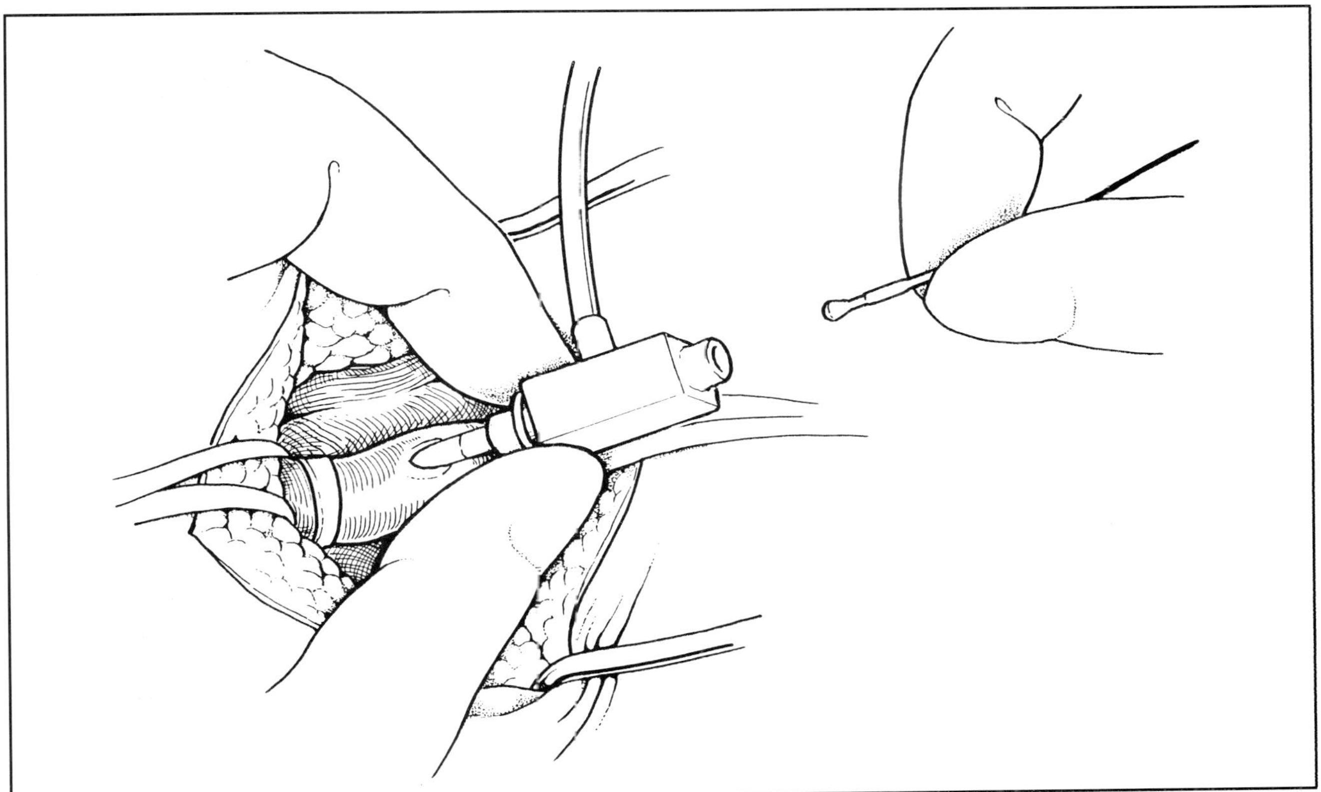

Fig. 77. A 2.5-mm diameter laser probe is inserted into the lumen through the sheath.

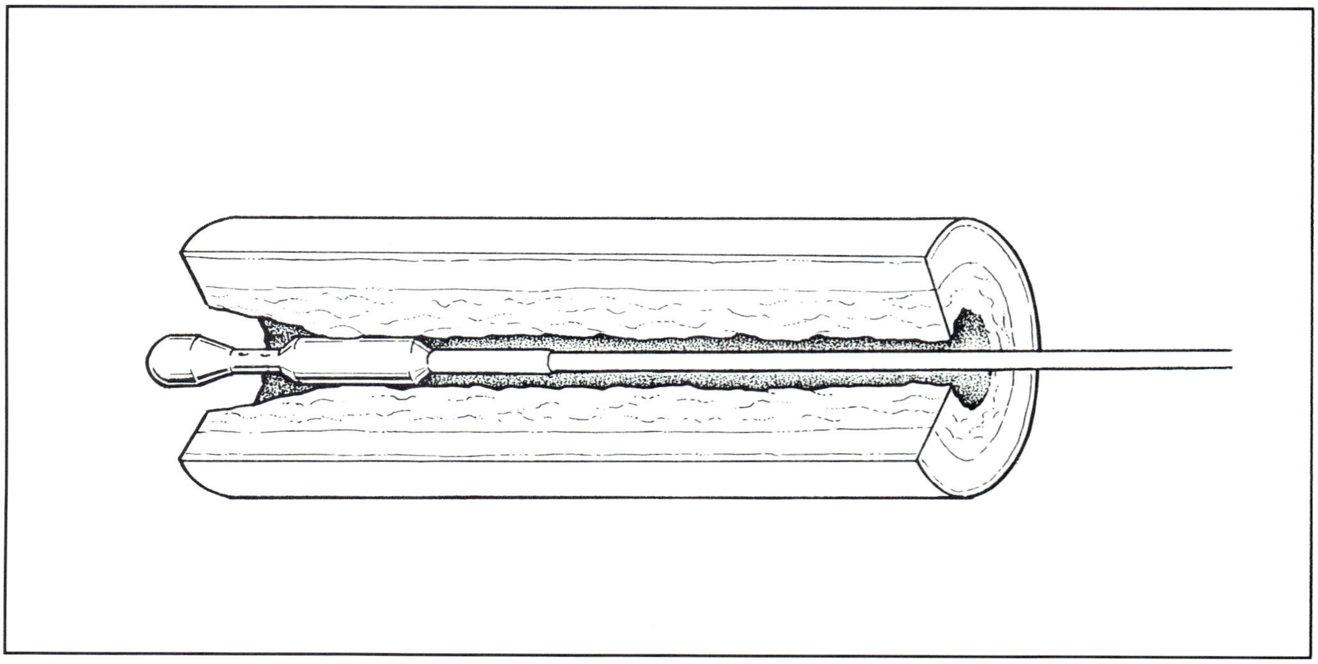

Fig. 78a

The probe is activated and advanced in a back-and-forth motion under fluoroscopy throughout the lesion (Fig. 78a and b).

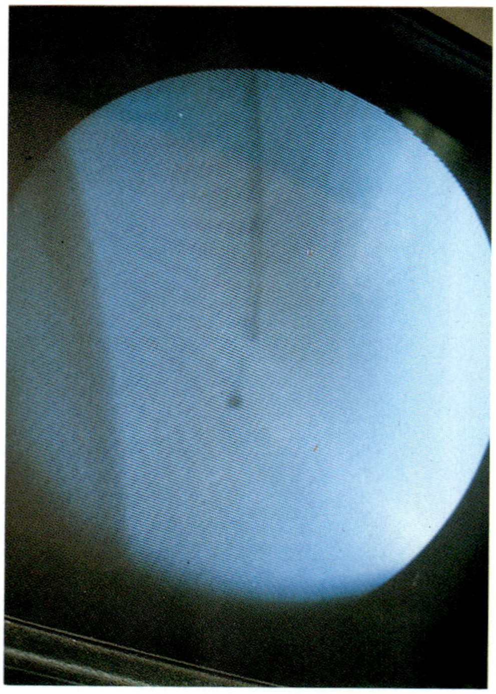

Fig. 78b

While advancing the laser probe, contrast dye is periodically injected to evaluate the new path and detect possible complications.

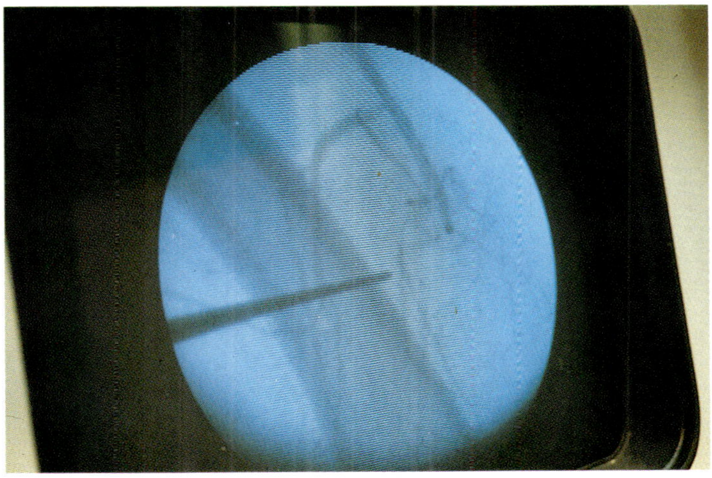

Fig. 79

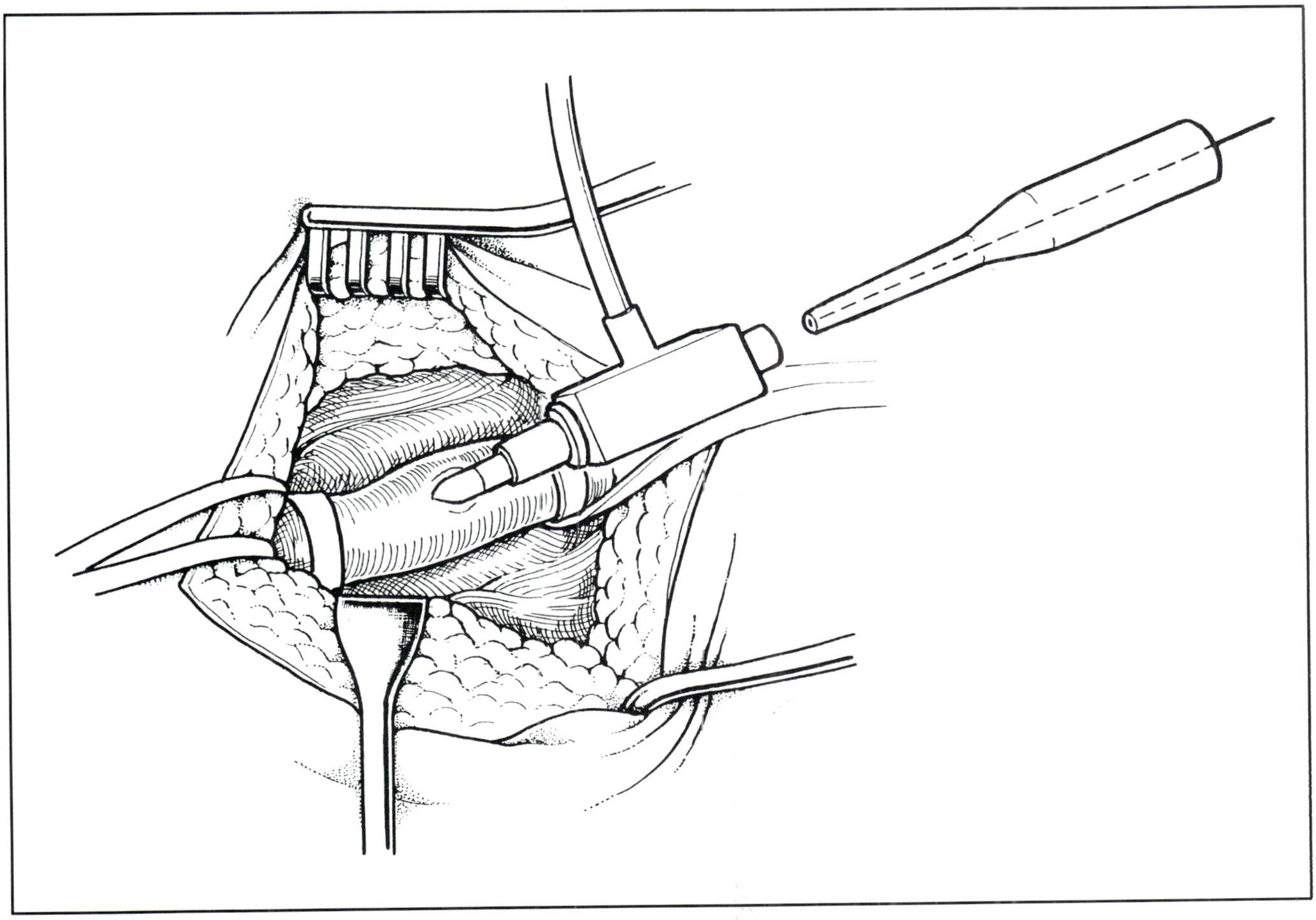

Fig. 80. A completion arteriogram should be performed on all patients to assess success, as well as to detect possible complications. After creation of a new channel, the hydrophilic guidewire is replaced into the lumen.

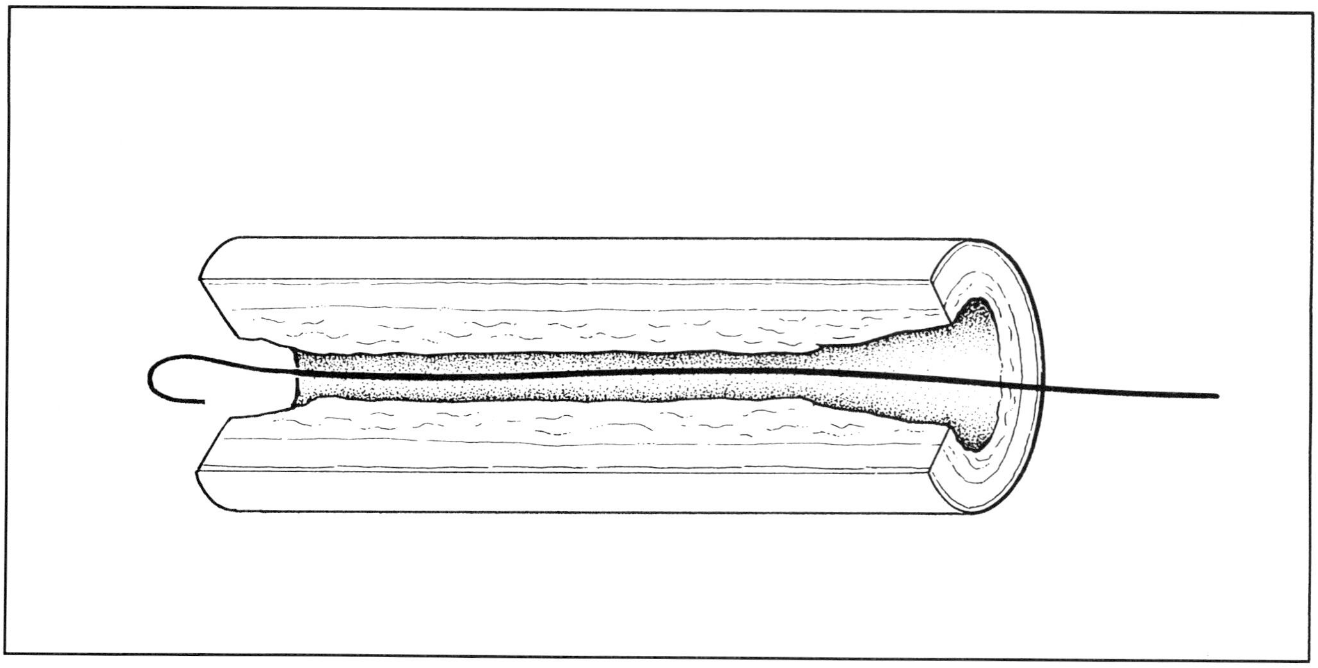

Fig. 81. The hydrophilic guidewire is advanced distally through the newly created channel to facilitate further procedures such as balloon dilatation (see chapter V).

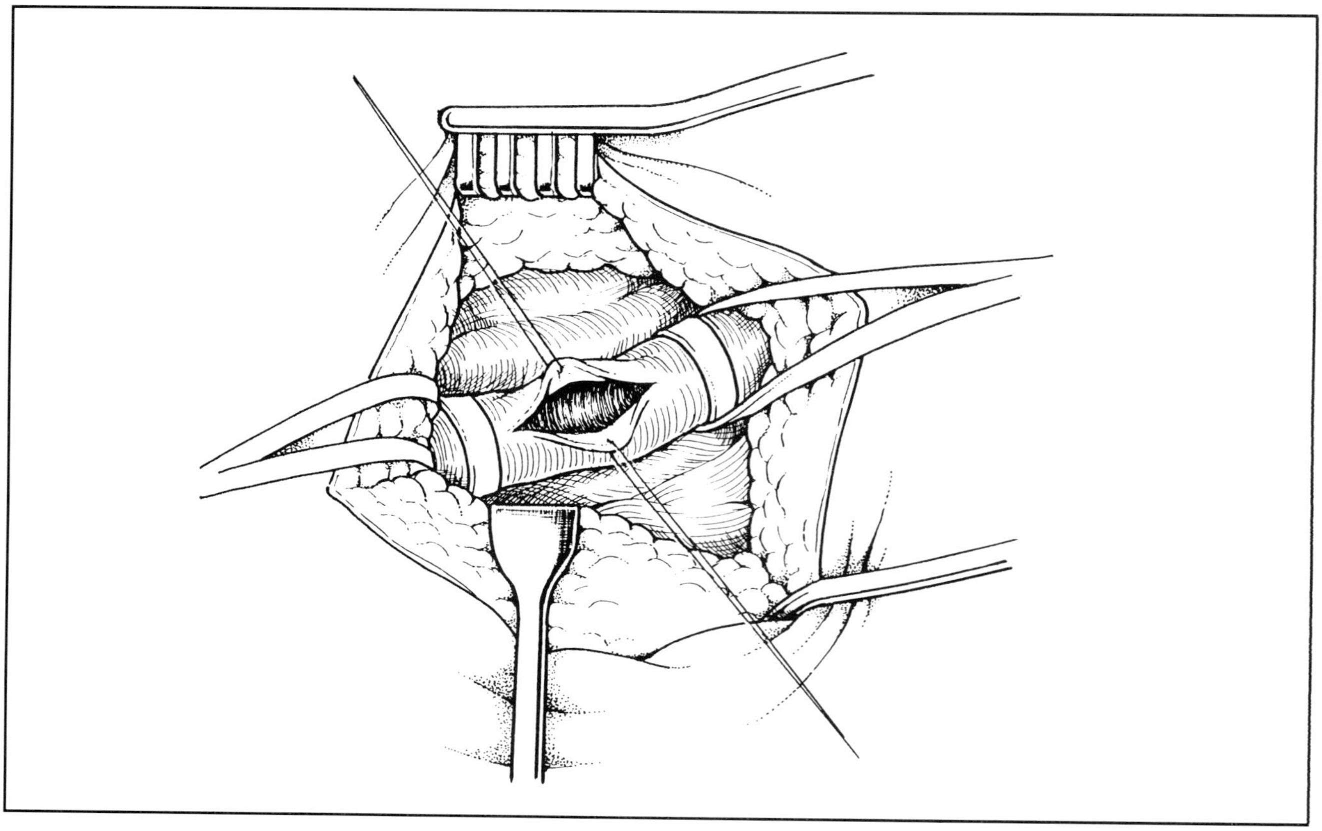

Fig. 82. After exposure of the CFA, arteriotomy is performed if the artery is markedly hard and shrunk with complete occlusion.

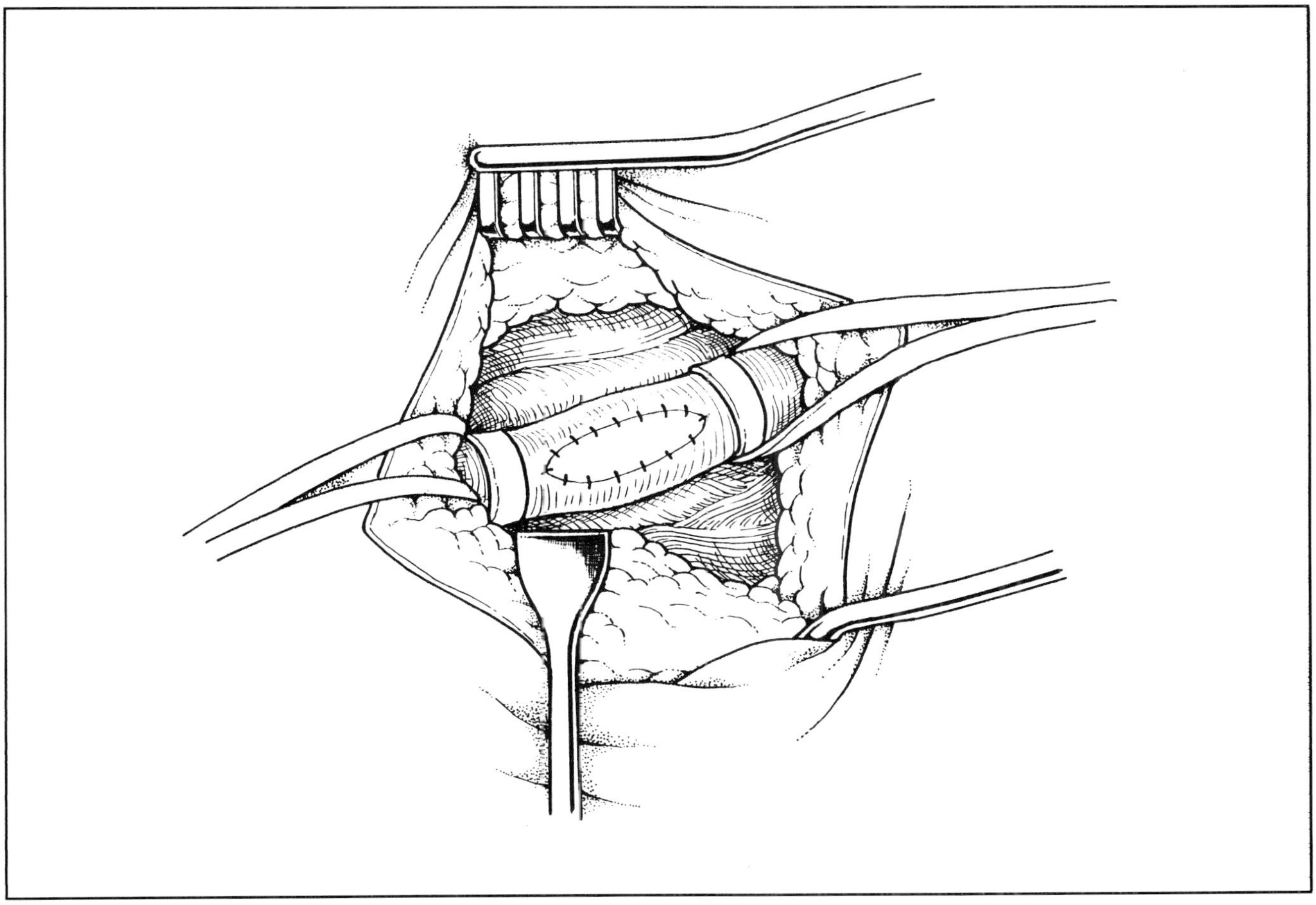

Fig. 83. Insertion techniques for the French introducer sheath, a hydrophilic guide wire and laser probes are the same as described in this chapter. After the angioplasty, the arteriotomy is closed with a vein patch.

Complications of the Surgical Approach

1. Wound infection
2. Pseudoaneurysm formation
3. Hematoma at the incision site
4. Extravasation of contrast media from arteriotomy site

Chapter 5

LASER-ASSISTED BALLOON ANGIOPLASTY (LABA)

Laser energy is used successfully in the ablation of plaques in peripheral arteries. However, the laser recanalization (the new channel) may not be adequate in respect to arterial size as well as blood flow. In such cases, a further adjunctive procedure is needed to enlarge the newly created narrow channel. Balloon dilatation is effective in accomplishing adequate dilatation of the narrower channels. Thus, laser recanalization must be followed by balloon dilatation in such cases at the same time unless and until larger probes are available.

Indications for Laser-Assisted Balloon Angioplasty (LABA)

1. Inadequate luminal diameter after successful laser recanalization
2. Intima dissection during lasing (Chapter VII)

Procedure

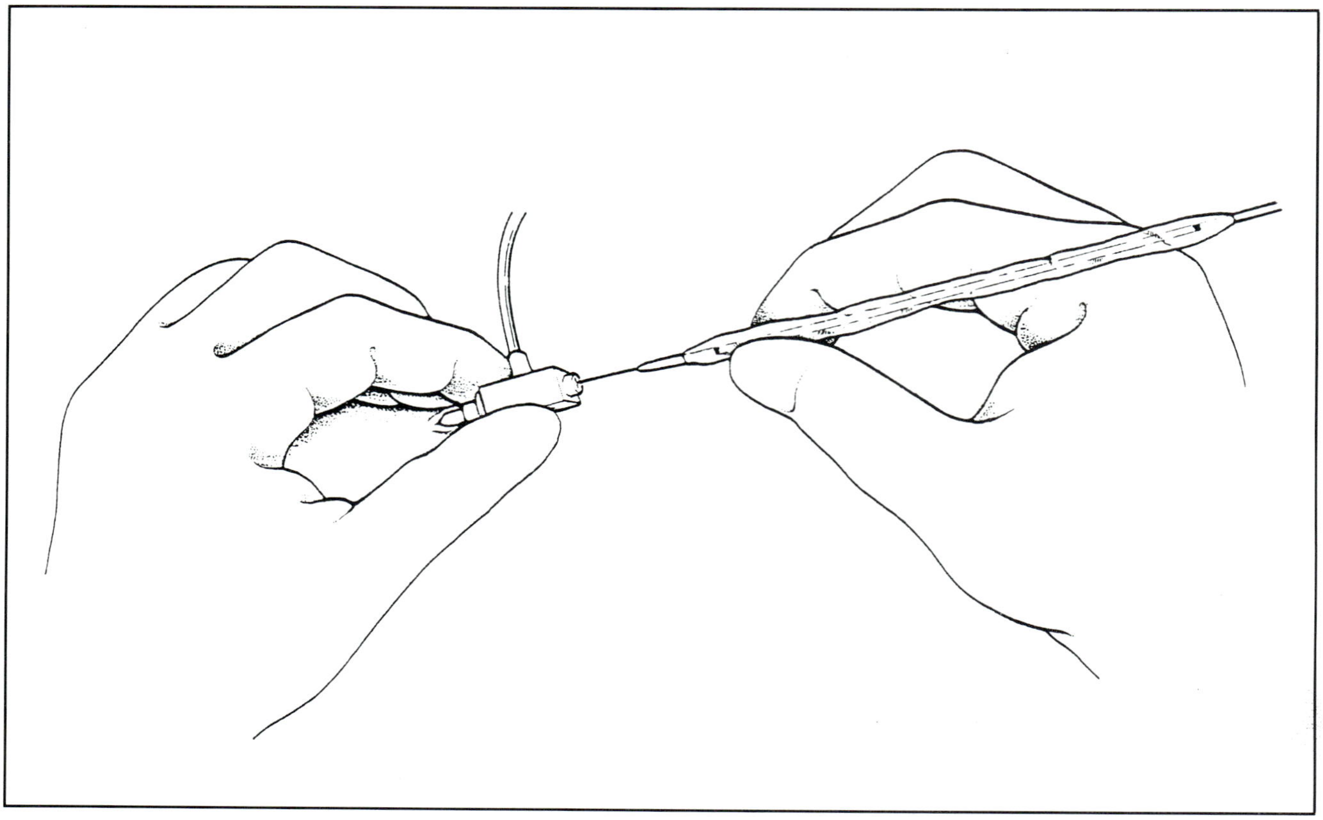

Fig. 84a

Laser recanalization using a 2.5-mm tipped laser probe should be performed as described in Chapters II and III. The hydrophilic guidewire is advanced and passed through the newly created channel. A balloon catheter (Gruentzig or Olbert) is then slipped over the guidewire (Fig. 84a and b).

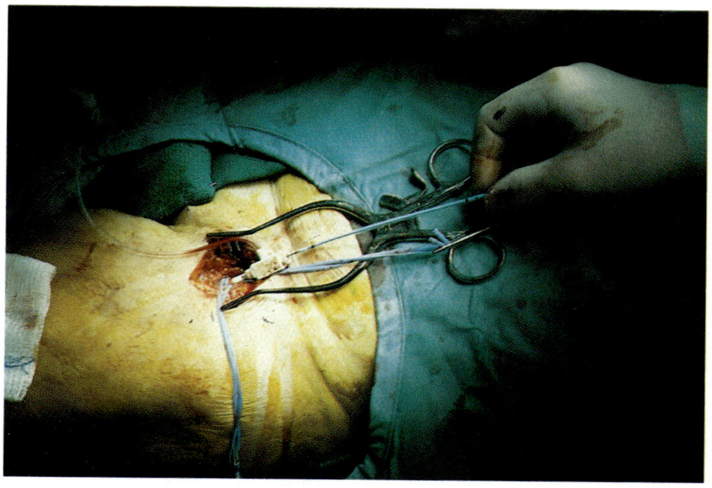

Fig. 84b

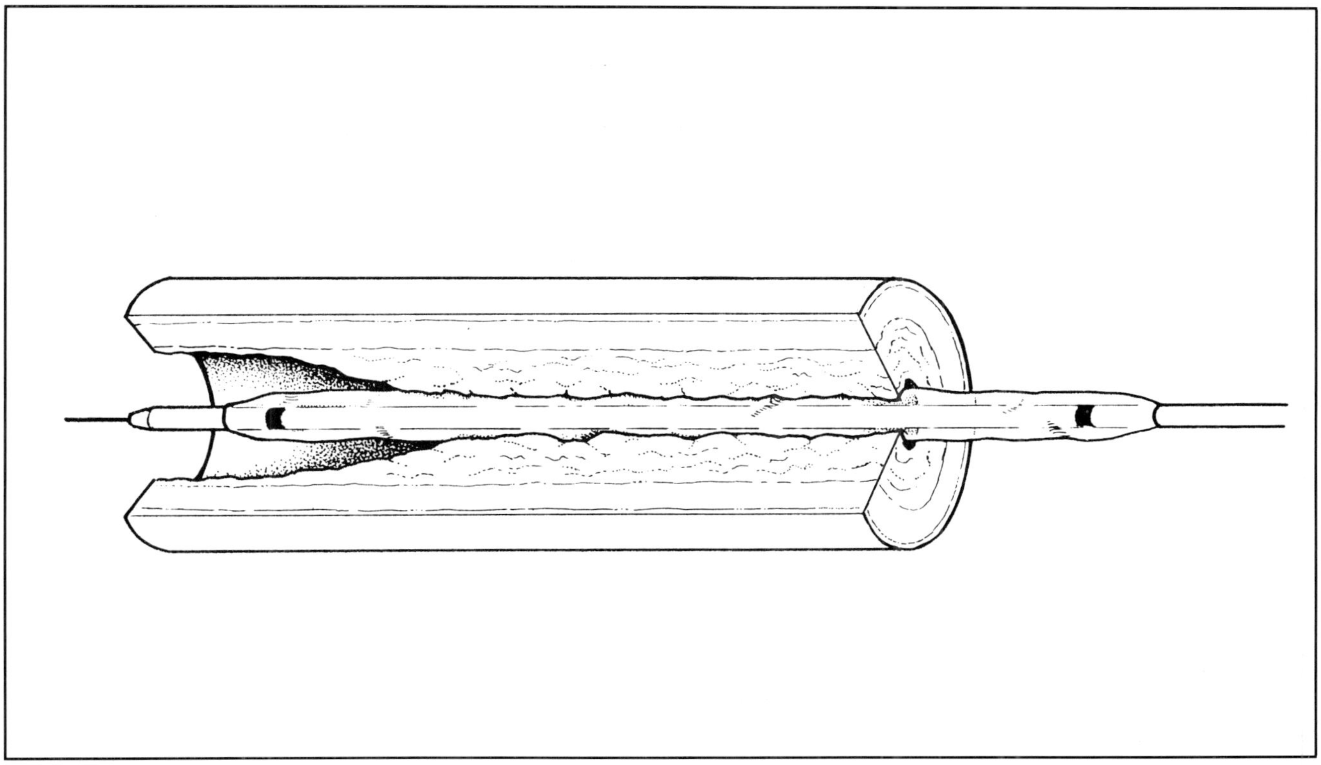

Fig. 85. The balloon catheter is advanced into the new channel.

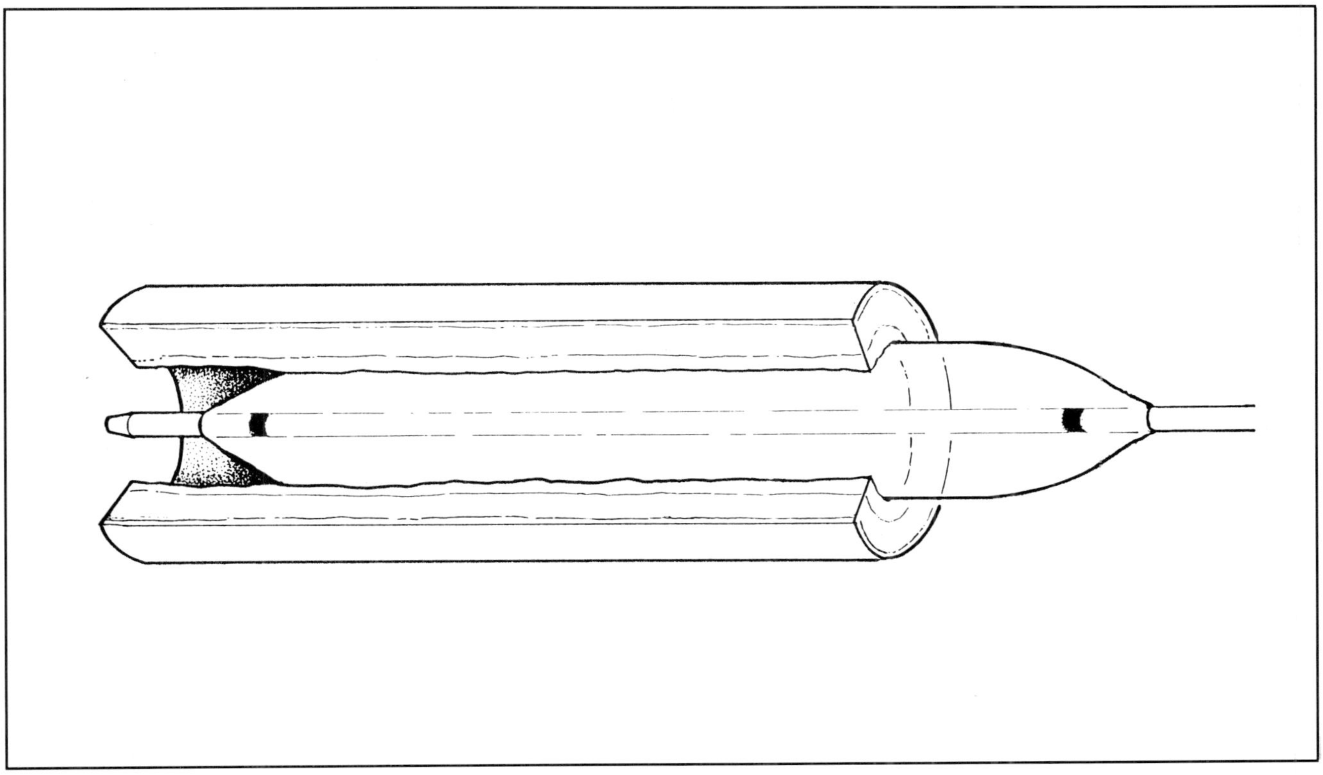

Fig. 86a

The balloon is then inflated (Fig. 86a and b).

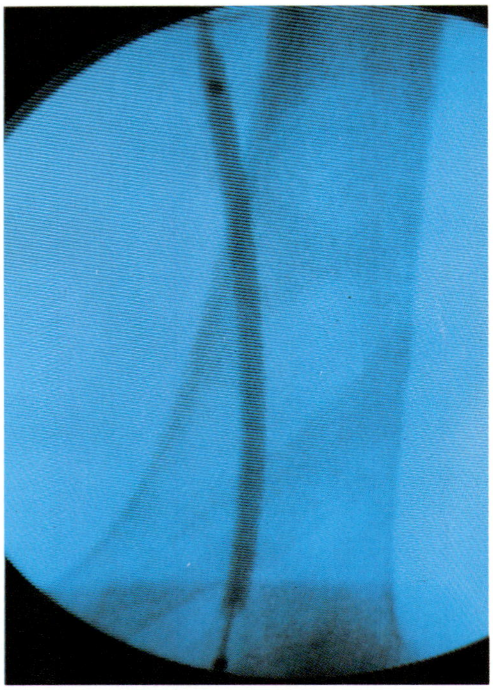

Fig. 86b

Using the Leveen inflator.

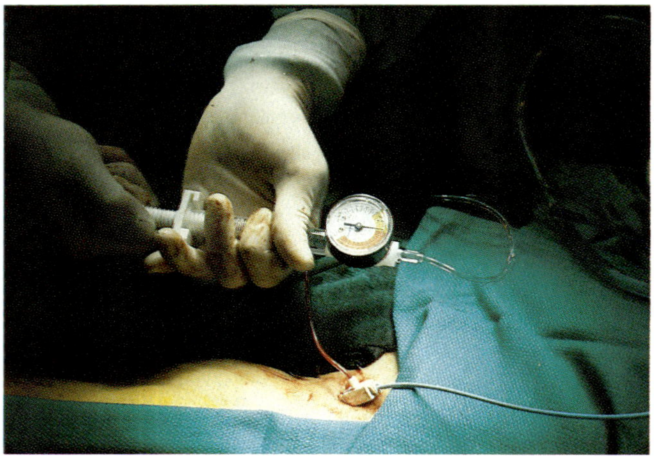

Fig. 87a

The Indeflator Plus.

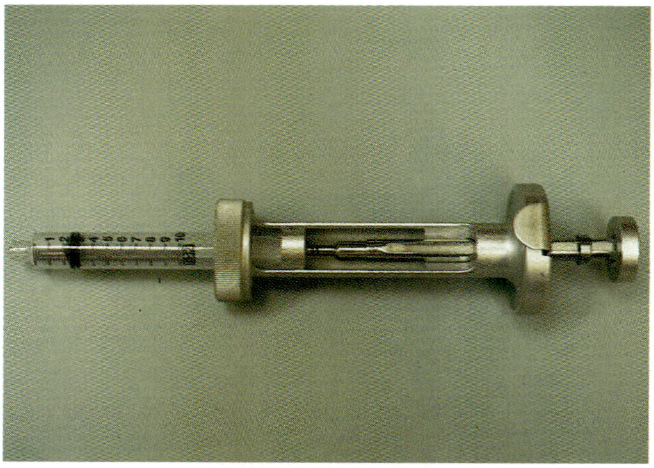

Fig. 87b

An appropriate pressure is maintained for two minutes. The proximal mark of the balloon is identified and marked using a needle stick in the skin. The balloon is deflated and pulled back until the lower mark comes to the site where the needle is stuck.

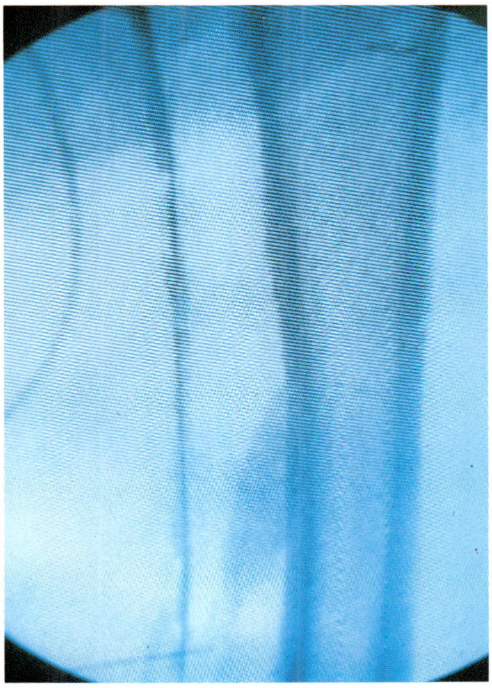

Fig. 88

This procedure is repeated throughout the channel under fluoroscopic observation. Adequate luminal size is confirmed by a completion arteriogram.

Complications

1. Bursting of the arterial wall (in case of balloon-artery size discrepancy)
2. Denuding of the arterial intima due to movement of an inflated balloon.

Chapter 6

LASER ANGIOPLASTY (LA)

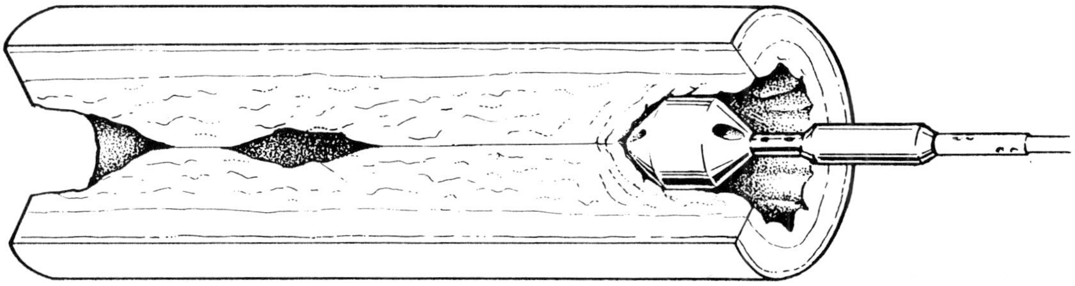

Fig. 89. Laser angioplasty is defined as the application of progressively larger-diameter laser probes to create an adequate arterial channel. A first attempt with a large-diameter (4.2-mm) laser probe would result in clogging of the arterial lumen with an atheromatous plaque rather than creating a big channel.

Recanalization, therefore, should start with a small-diameter laser tip (2.5-mm), and continue with progressively larger-diameter tips (3.5-, 4.2-, 5.0-mm) according to the arterial lumen to thus creating an adequate blood flow.

Laser recanalization using a small laser tip (2.5-mm) may not be adequate in large-diameter arteries such as the SFA; therefore, either balloon dilatation or further ablation using larger laser tips in the channel becomes mandatory. Thus, laser angioplasty may prove to be a substitute for laser-assisted balloon angioplasty, especially because the former ablates the occluded plaque and patency may last longer; however, further evaluation is needed. As with the balloon, extra precautions are necessary in selecting the appropriate size of laser tip that correlates with arterial size. Currently, the available number of different-sized laser tips is limited. A gradual increment of 0.1-mm diameter laser tips will improve the technology in vascular surgery.

Indications for Laser Angioplasty (LA)

1. Large artery
2. Narrow channel
3. Successful laser recanalization

Procedure for Laser Angioplasty (LA)

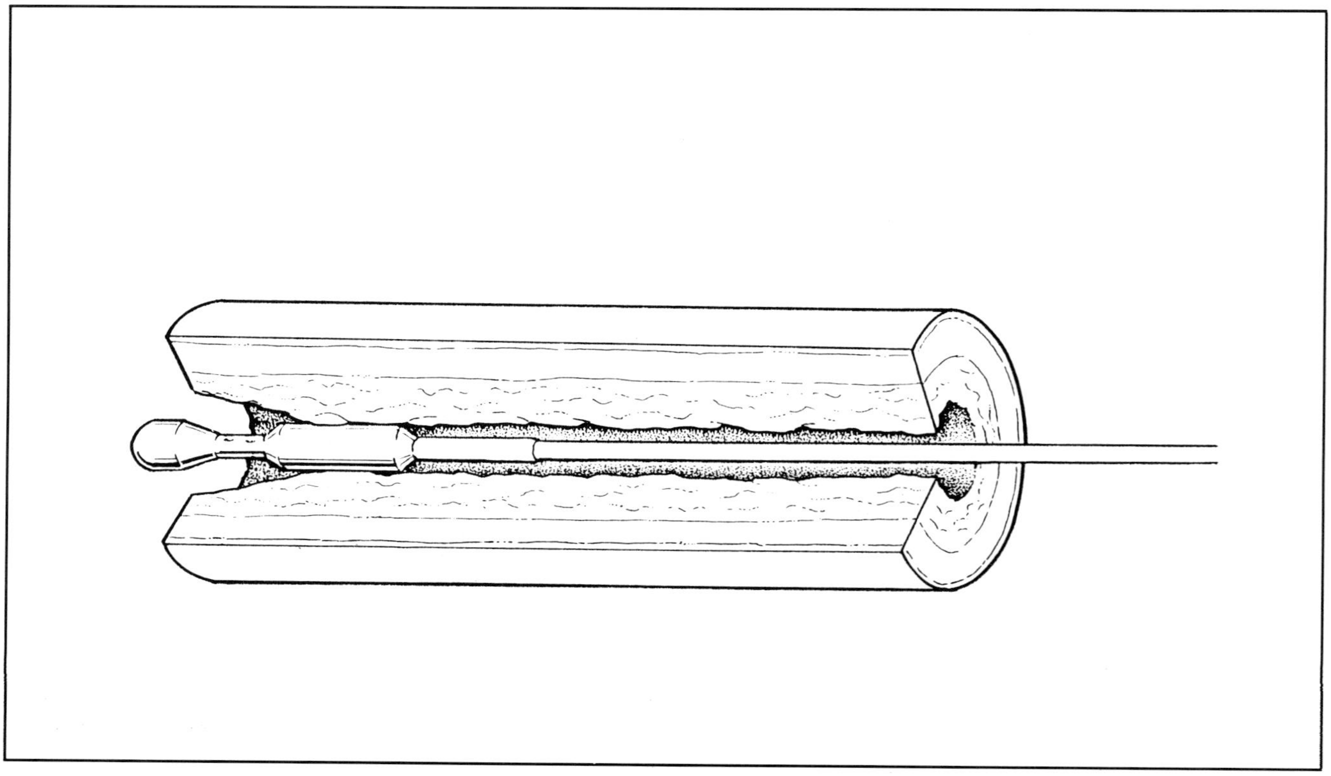

Fig. 90. A 2.5-mm diameter tipped laser probe is used for creation of a new channel in an occlusive lesion.

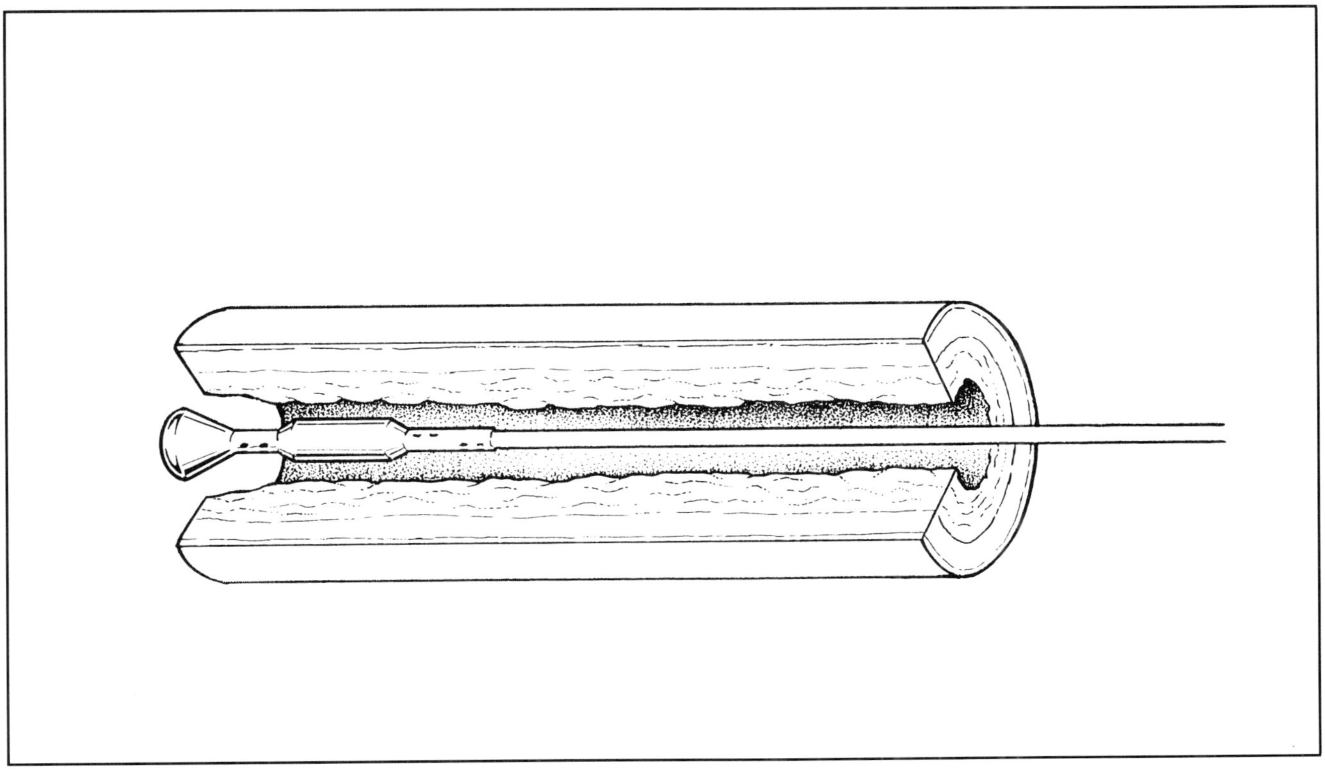

Fig. 91. Subsequently, a 3.5-mm laser probe expands the channel created by the 2.5-mm probe.

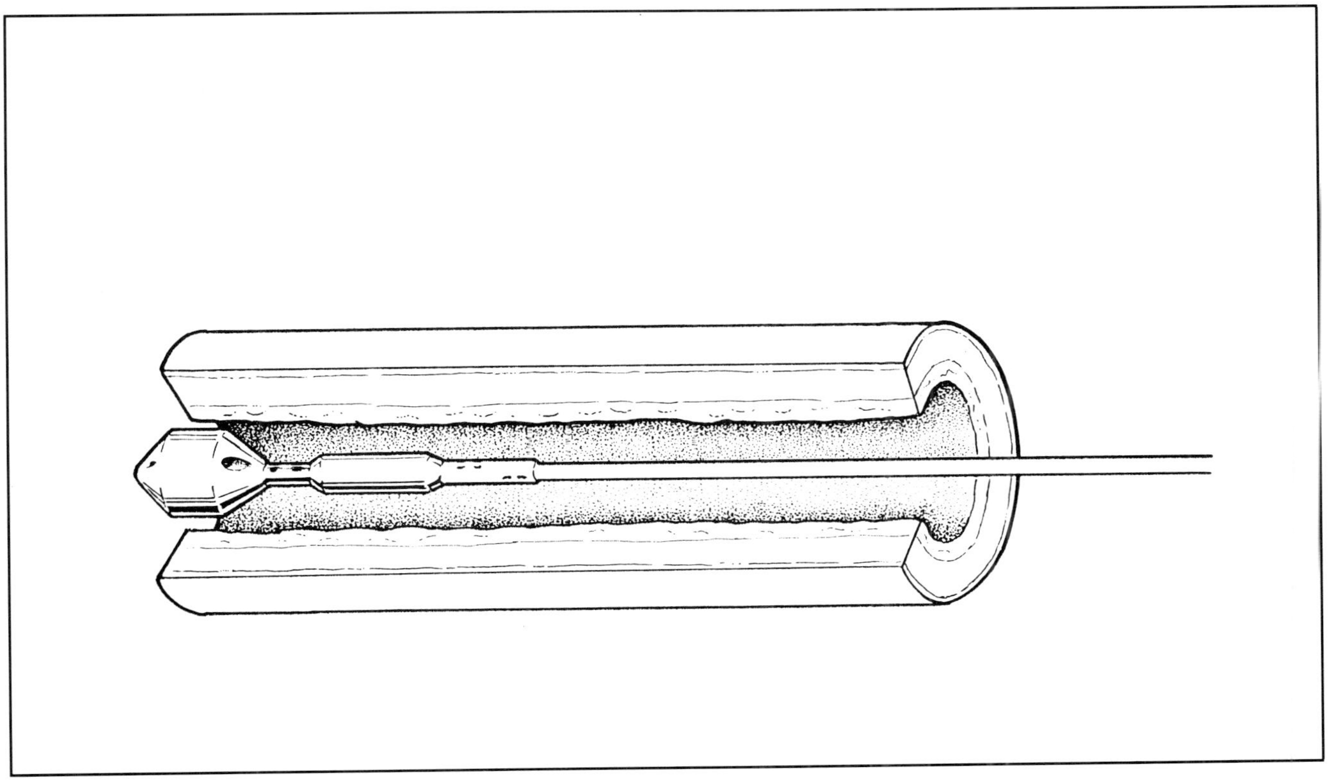

Fig. 92. If needed, further ablation may be done using a 4.2-mm diameter laser tip.

Complications of LA

1. Perforation of arterial wall
2. Weakening of arterial wall
3. Aneurysm formation

Chapter 7
LASER COMPLICATIONS

Acute Complications

Intima Dissection

The arterial intima can be torn mechanically by the laser probe and also by a guidewire or balloon catheter. The intimal dissection can be detected immediately under fluoroscopy using contrast media. An arteriogram of the intimal dissection will show thin and longitudinal slit-like pooling of retained contrast media near the arterial lumen. The intimal dissection can be corrected by a balloon dilatation.

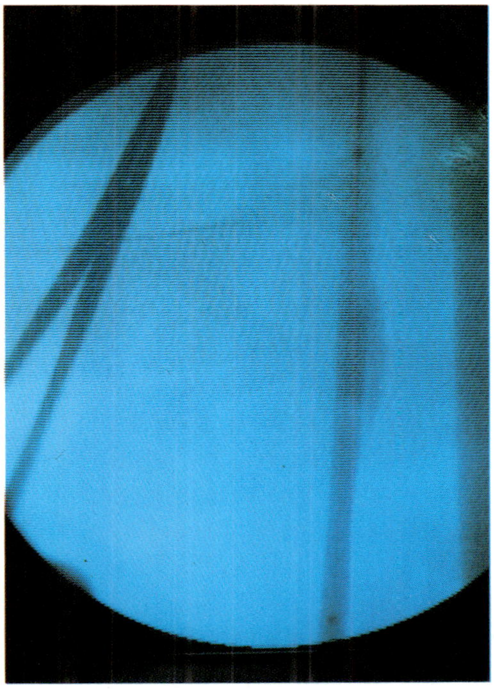

Fig. 93

Arterial wall perforation

Arterial wall perforation is a major complication observed in laser recanalization. Occurrence of this complication is primarily associated with the length as well as consistency of occlusion. In other words, arterial wall perforation is most often noted in recanalization of total-length occlusions and hard atheromatous (densely calcified) lesions. It is promptly detected under fluroscope by observing extravasation of the contrast medium.

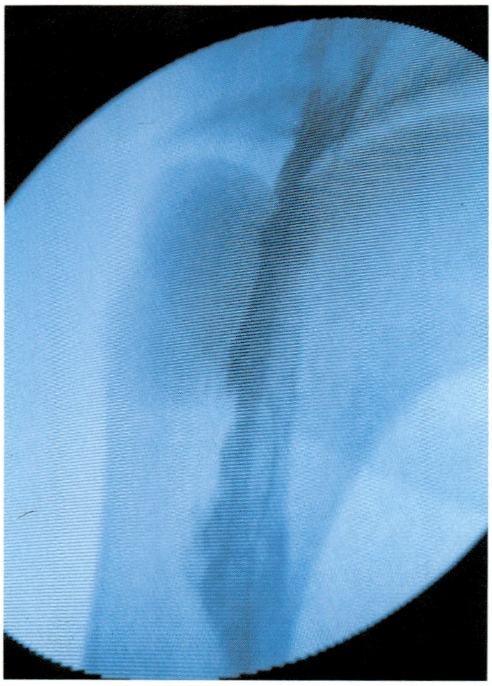

Fig. 94

Gentle advancement of the laser probe and fluoroscopic confirmation will prevent this complication. The perforation is treated by ligating the artery proximal to the perforation and then directly repairing the perforated arterial wall. Further management depends upon the location and nature of the perforation. In some cases, an appropriate reconstructive bypass surgery is required. Shown here is a right femoral-popliteal bypass.

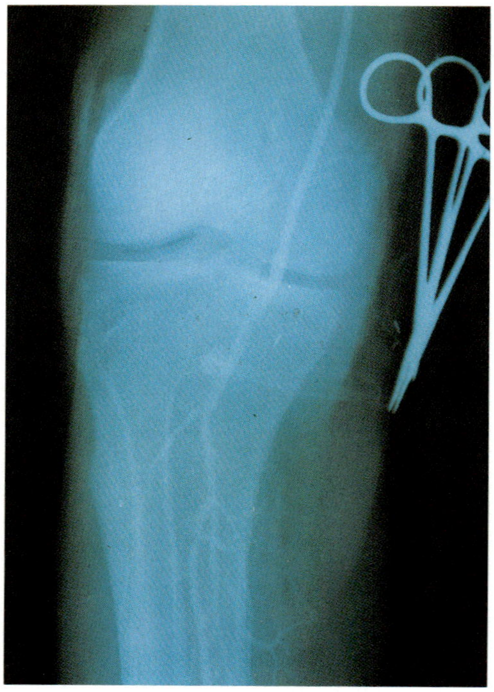

Fig. 95

Total-length occlusion of the SFA.

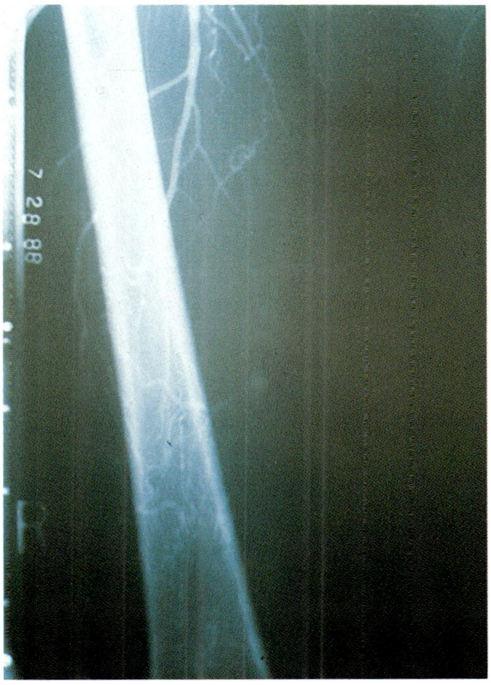

Fig. 96

Embolization in distal artery

Laser recanalization can cause acute embolization of the distal arteries, but this can be avoided by arteriotomy and open technique (after clamping proximal and distal ends of the arteriotomy, declamping the distal only allows that distal blood flows retrogradely and pushes out the embolus from the arteriotomy).

Chronic Complications

Thrombus formation

The heated laser probe can damage the arterial intima; platelets then aggregate and thrombus formation occurs. Administration of antiplatelet drugs, therefore is recommended after laser treatment.

Pseudoaneurysm formation

Pseudoaneurysm may occur with a percutaneous approach. This problem can be avoided by compression of the groin for 30 minutes after the procedure.

Chapter 8

LIMITATIONS OF LASER TREATMENT

Extent of Lesion

Table 7 shows immediate results of Argon and Nd:YAG laser in our study. In tight stenoses and segmental occlusions, laser recanalization is quite successful; however, in longer occlusions more than 20 cm, the success rate decreases markedly. Such occlusion, therefore, is not an appropriate indication for currently available laser applications.

Table 7. Immediate results of laser arterial reconstruction in 203 legs.

		No. of legs				
			Successful angioplasty (recanalized to adequate diameter)		Unsuccessful angioplasty	
Type of lesion	*Type of laser*	*Total*	*LR*	*LR + BD (LABA)*	*Too narrow recanalization*	*Impossible recanalization*
Stenosis	Argon	5	2 (40%)	0	3 (60%)	0
	YAG	16	4 (25%)	10 (63%)	2 (13%)	0
		21	5 (29%)	10 (47%)	5 (24%)	0
Segmental occlusion	Argon	45	27 (60%)	0	10 (22%)	8 (18%)
	YAG	63	3 (5%)	36 (57%)	6 (10%)	18 (29%)
		108	30 (28%)	36 (33%)	16 (15%)	26 (24%)
Total-length occlusion	Argon	24	0	0	7 (29%)	17 (71%)
	YAG	31	1 (3%)	16 (52%)	0	14 (45%)
		55	1 (2%)	16 (29%)	7 (13%)	31 (56%)
Graft occlusion	Argon	15	15 (100%)	0	0	0
	YAG	4	3 (75%)	0	0	1 (25%)
		19	18 (95%)	0	0	1 (5%)
Total		203	55 (27%)	62 (31%)	28 (14%)	58 (29%)

LR, laser recanalization; BD, balloon dilation; LABA, laser-assisted balloon angioplasty
*Statistically significant difference between the success rate of total-length occlusion and that of others ($p < 0.001$)

Characteristics of Lesion

Table 8 shows the immediate results obtained with total-length occlusions of the SFA and PA, according to the degree of calcification.[73] In the case of soft atherosclerosis with small arterial lumen, the laser recanalization rate was reasonable, while in the case of hard atherosclerosis without arterial lumen on intraoperative arteriogram (advanced atherosclerosis), the recanalization rate was very poor. Thus, the occlusions 20 cm or longer having advanced atherosclerosis, the laser was unsuccessful.

Table 8. Immediate operative results of total-length occlusion of SFA and popliteal artery (PA) in relation to degree of calcification.[73]

			No. of legs			
				Successful angioplasty (recanalized to adequate diameter)	Unsuccessful angioplasty	
Degree of calcification	*Artery*	*Type of laser*	*Total*		*Too narrow recanalization*	*Impossible recanalization*
Soft atherosclerosis with some evidence of limited arterial lumen*	SFA	Argon	7	0	5 (71%)	2 (29%)
		YAG	1	0		1 (100%)
	PA	Argon	0	0	0	0
		YAG	3	3 (100%)	0	0
			11	3 (27%)	5 (46%)	3 (27%)
Hard atherosclerosis without any evidence of lumen*	SFA	Argon	16	0	2 (13%)	14 (87%)
		YAG	6	0	0	6 (100%)
	PA	Argon	1	0	0	1 (100%)
		YAG	2	0		2 (100%)
			25	0	2 (8%)	23 (92%)

*There was a statistically significant difference of recanalization rate between groups

Chapter 9

SELECTED CASE STUDIES

Tight Stenosis of the SFA (Laser-Assisted Balloon Angioplasty)

A 70-year-old man had been suffering from incapacitating intermittent claudication in his right leg for six months. He had no history of rest pain or tissue loss. An arteriogram showed a tight stenosis in the distal 20-cm of the right SFA.

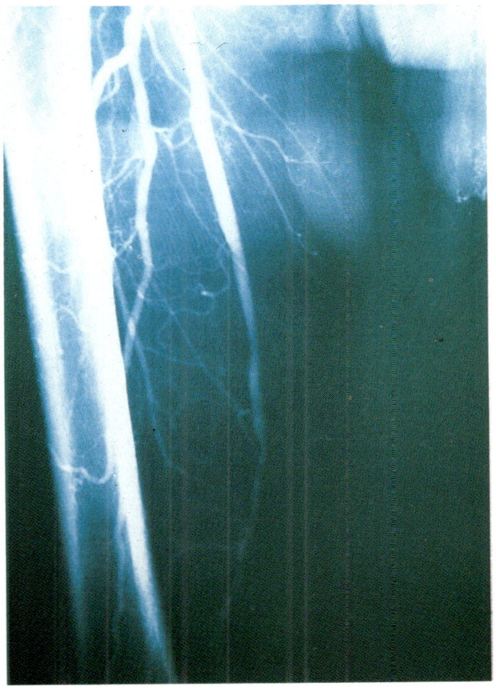

Fig. 97

The preoperative ankle brachial index (ABI) of the leg was 0.75. A percutaneous approach was used. A guidewire was attempted, but could not pass through the lesion. Subsequently, a 2.5-mm laser probe was activated at 15 watts and advanced to recanalize the lesion. A total of 448 joules was required to create a new lumen,

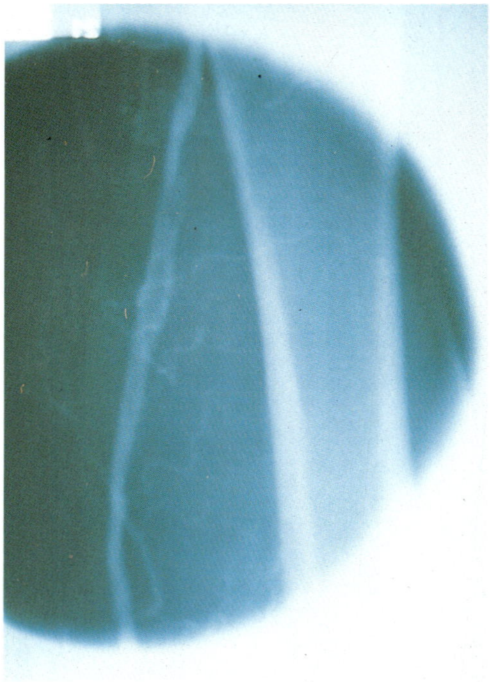

Fig. 98

. . . but the new lumen was inadequate and balloon dilatation was performed. After the procedure, the ABI was 0.9.

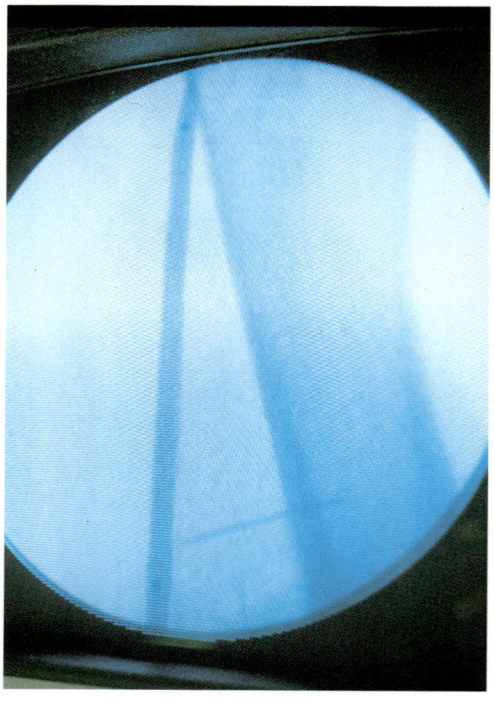

Fig. 99

Segmental occlusion of the Superficial Femoral Artery (SFA)

Proximal Occlusion

Laser-Assisted Balloon Angioplasty

A 60-year-old man came to the office complaining of incapacitating intermittent claudication at a distance of 1/2 block. The patient had had these symptoms for two years. An arteriogram showed complete occlusion of the left proximal SFA (20-cm in length).

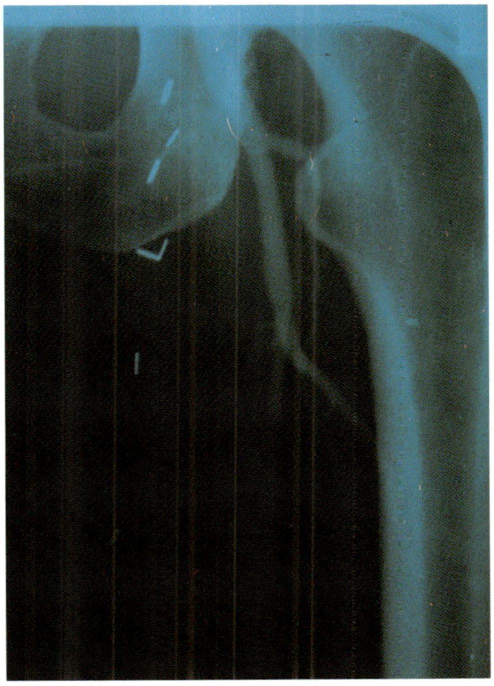

Fig. 100

The distal SFA, popliteal and tibial arteries were patent. ABI in the left leg was 0.47. A cut-down approach was used. A guidewire was attempted but failed to pass through the lesion. A 2.5-mm diameter tipped laser probe (14 watts) was used to create a new channel and successfully passed through the lesion at a total energy of 175 joules. An activated 3.5-mm diameter tipped laser probe was then used to create a larger lumen and successfully passed through the lesion at a total energy of 177 joules.

The diameter of the newly created channel using the 3.5-mm probe, however, was still inadequate; therefore, a balloon dilatation was then performed. Postprocedural ABI of 1.0 was achieved in the leg.

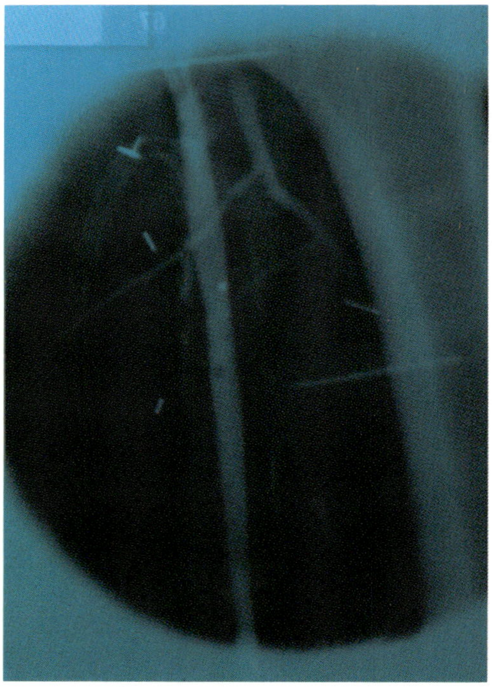

Fig. 101

Midportion Occlusion

Laser-Assisted Balloon Angioplasty

A 62-year-old women was admitted complaining of rest pain in her left leg. A preoperative arteriogram revealed complete occlusion of the left middle SFA (20-cm in length).

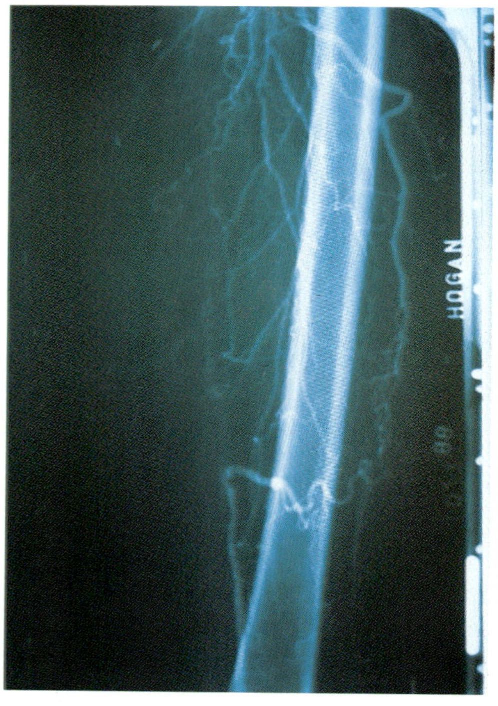

Fig. 102

Both the proximal and distal SFA were patent but stenotic. Distally, only the peroneal artery was patent. The Doppler examination disclosed 0.0 ABI. A cut-down was done and a guidewire could not pass through the lesion. A 2.5-mm diameter tipped laser probe was used at 15 watts and the occlusion was successfully recanalized at 410 joules. The newly created lumen was inadequate, however, and subsequently a balloon dilatation was required. After the procedure, the ABI was 0.4.

Fig. 103

Distal Occlusion

Laser-Assisted Balloon Angioplasty

A 55-year-old man had incapacitating intermittent claudication in his right leg at a distance of one block. The patient had had the symptoms for three years. An arteriogram revealed a 6.5-cm occlusion in the right distal SFA.

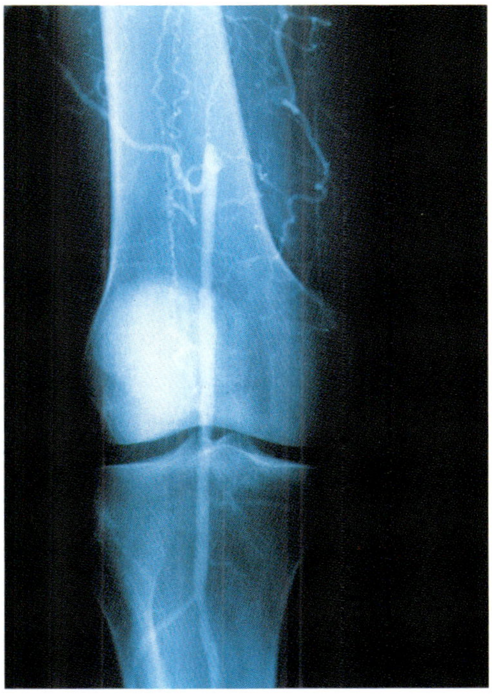

Fig. 104

Right proximal SFA and PA were stenotic, but the tibial arteries were patent. The ABI of the right leg was 0.44. A percutaneous approach was done and the guidewire could not pass through the lesion. A 2.5-mm tipped laser probe successfully ablated the atheromatous plaque at 147 joules. Because the newly created lumen was not adequate, a balloon dilatation was done and adequate lumen was obtained. Postprocedural ABI was 0.92.

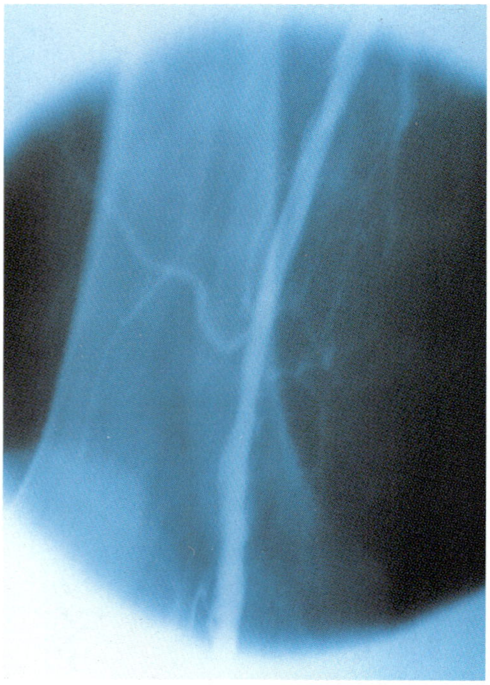

Fig. 105

Total Length Occlusion of the SFA

Bypass Surgery

A 43-year-old man had symptoms of incapacitating intermittent claudication at a distance of one block in his right leg for five years. He had no rest pain and tissue loss. An arteriogram revealed total-length occlusion of the right SFA.

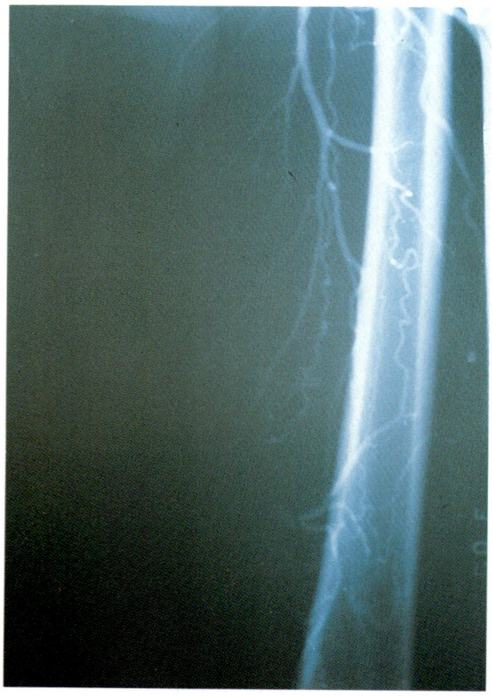

Fig. 106

Distally, the anterior tibial artery was completely occluded but the peroneal and posterior tibial arteries were patent.

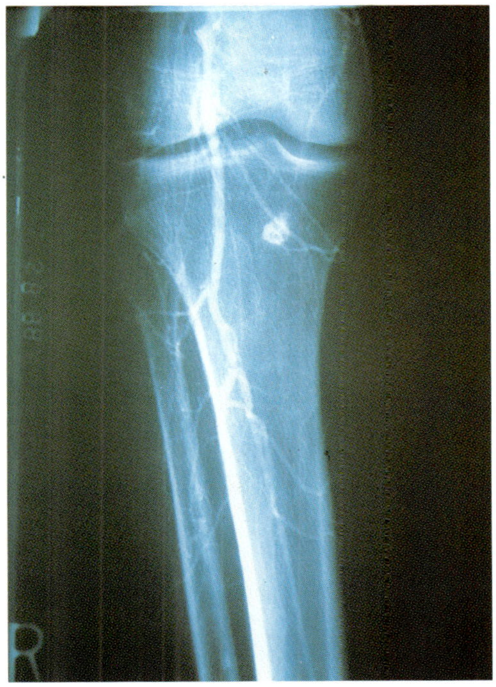

Fig. 107

The ABI of the leg was 0.56. A cut-down approach was used and the guidewire did pass through the lesion. A 2.5-mm diameter tipped laser probe was then passed both anterograde and retrograde. Although 1099 joules energy were used, a new channel could not be created in the occlusion; therefore, a femoral-popliteal bypass was performed using a reversed saphenous vein graft. Postoperative ABI was 0.83.

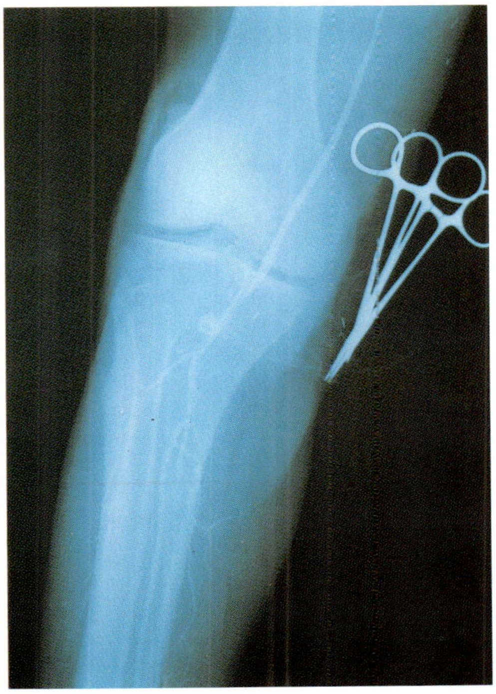

Fig. 108

Occlusive Lesion of the Popliteal Artery (PA)

Laser Angioplasty

A 64-year-old man had undergone left femoral-popliteal bypass which used a polytetrafluorethylene (PTFE) graft in April 1988 and had rest pain in his left leg two months after the surgery. Preoperative ABI was 0.52. An arteriogram showed complete occlusion of the popliteal artery.

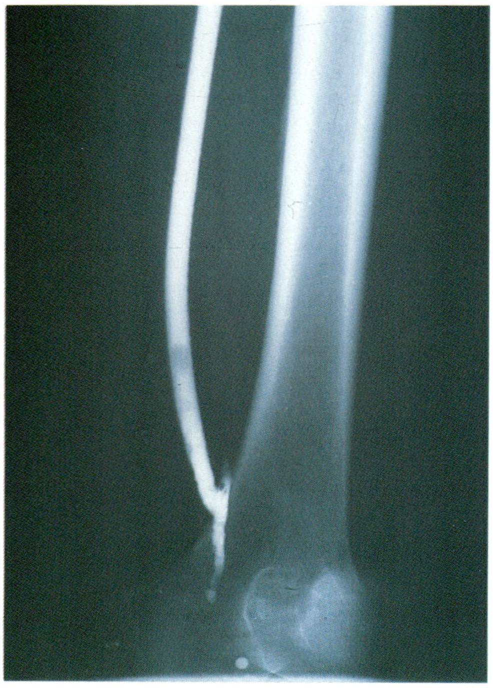

Fig. 109

Only the posterior tibial artery was patent distally. A cut-down approach was used. A guide-wire could not pass through the lesion. The 2.5-mm metalic laser tip created a new channel. A total of 211 joules were required for the creation of the channel. The ABI improved to 0.72 postoperatively.

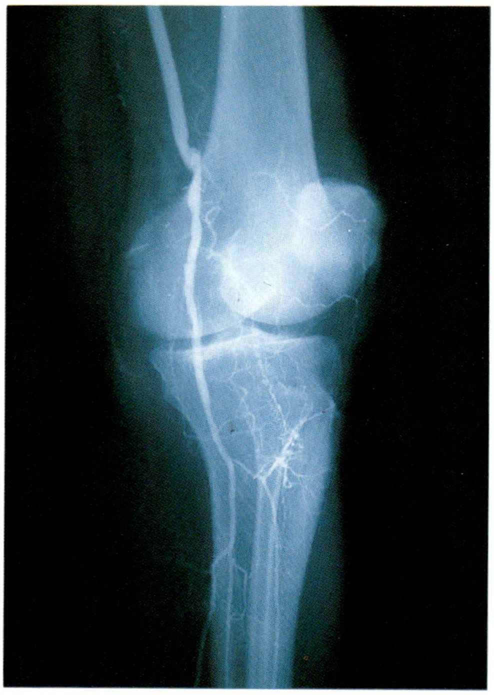

Fig. 110

Combined Lesions

Occlusions of the Superficial Femoral Artery (SFA) and Popliteal Artery (PA)

Laser-Assisted Balloon Angioplasty

A 60-year-old man with incapacitating intermittent claudication in his right leg came to the office. The Doppler examination was 0.53 ABI. The arteriogram of the right leg showed complete occlusions of the distal SFA (25-cm) and PA (10-cm).

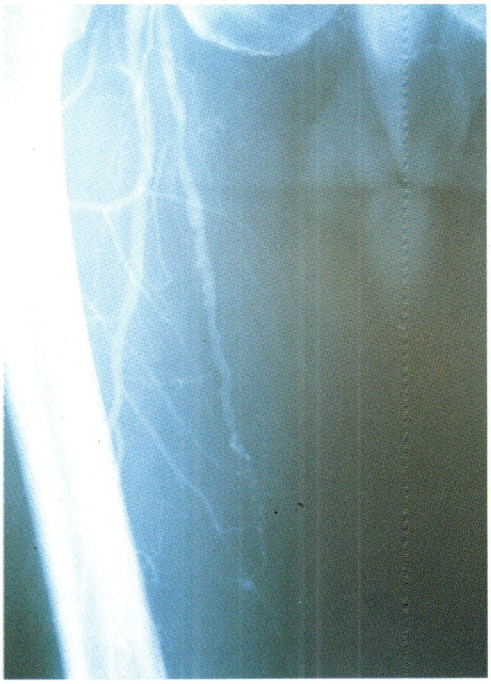

Fig. 111

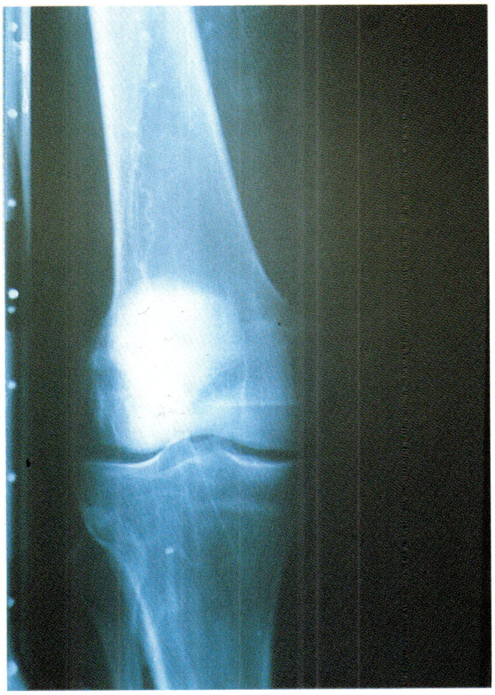

Fig. 112

A guidewire did not pass through the lesions. A 2.5-mm diameter tipped probe was successfully used at 261 joules to recanalize the lesion. Because the new channel was inadequate, a balloon dilatation was subsequently performed, and after the balloon dilatation, adequate luminal diameter was obtained. The ABI improved to 0.90.

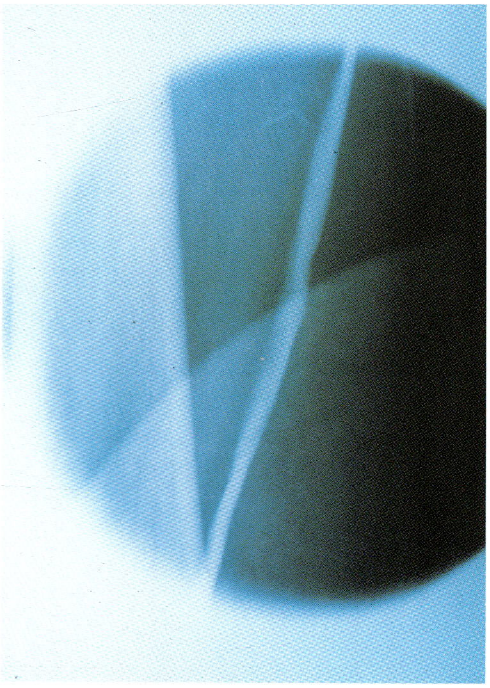

Fig. 113

Occlusions of the Superficial Femoral Artery Popliteal Artery and Tibial Arteries

(Proximal bypass with distal laser treatment)

A 64-year-old man presented with a gangrenous spot in his left toe. The ABI was 0.25 in the left leg. An arteriogram revealed total length occlusion of the left SFA . . .

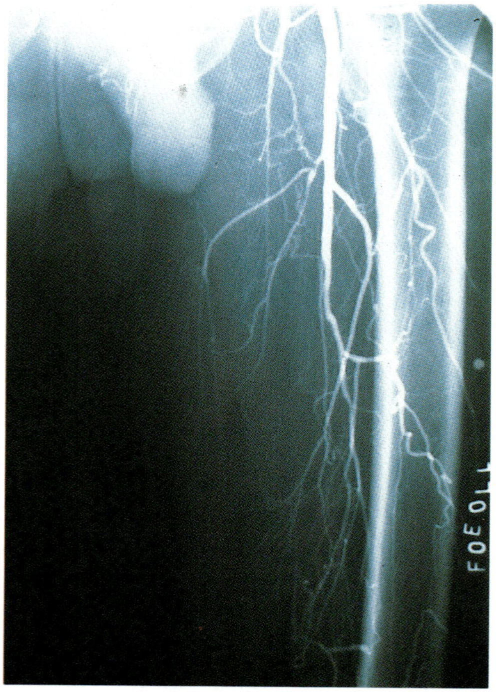

Fig. 114

and segmental occlusion of the PA and proximal posterior tibial artery.

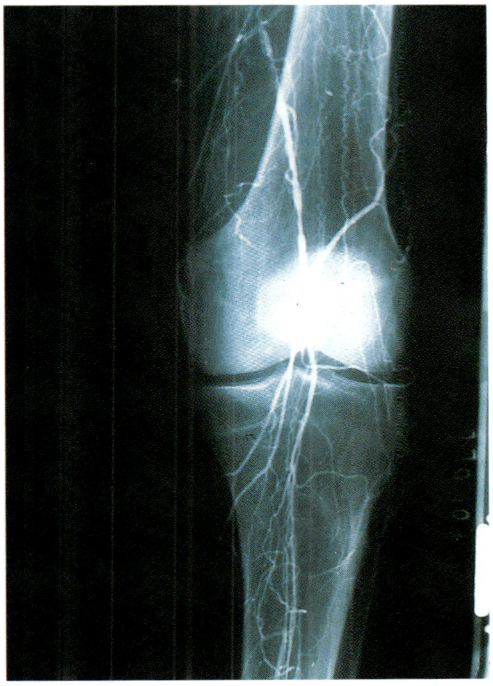

Fig. 115

The distal posterior tibial artery was patent.

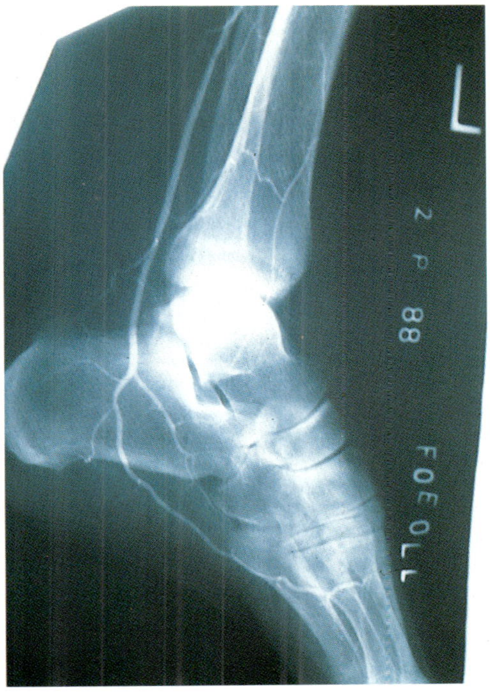

Fig. 116

A 1.5-mm diameter tipped laser probe passed through the proximal posterior tibial artery at a energy level of nine watts and a new channel was created with 61 joules; however, laser recanalization of the SFA and PA lesions was not successful. A femoral posterior tibial bypass was performed using saphenous vein *in situ*. Postoperative ABI was 0.92.

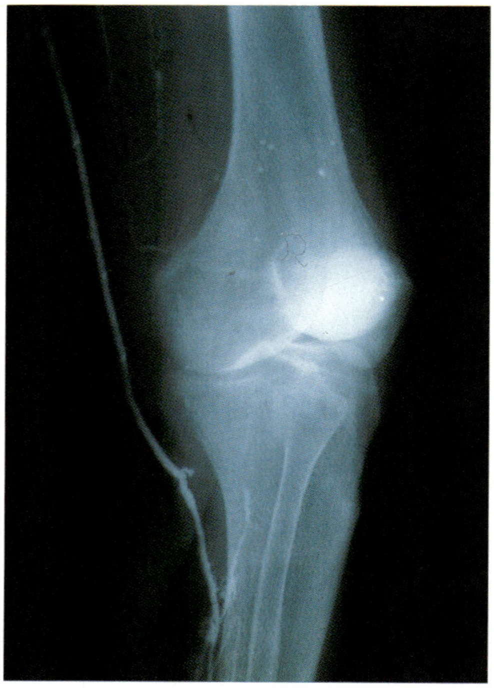

Fig. 117

Summary

Laser-assisted balloon angioplasty is a useful addition to the vascular surgeon's armamentarium. As data accumulates, however, certain limitations of this procedure have been recognized. Specifically, it has become clear that densely calcified atheromas cannot be evaporated and disobstructed, regardless of the type of laser used. In this situation, atherectomy also cannot be performed. In spite of this, for several reasons, LABA has a role to play in the practice of vascular surgery. First, though it is true that the majority of patients with vascular disease will still require bypass surgery, LABA may serve as an adjunct to bypass, allowing less complicated reconstructive procedures to be performed. In such patients, LABA and bypass can be performed at the same sitting in the operating room, necessitating a single anesthesia exposure. Second, in selected patients such as those at high risk due to concomitant medical conditions, LABA alone may still be the procedure of choice. Third, it is often difficult to determine if a lesion is amenable to LABA without attempting the procedure. Some complete occlusions on arteriogram are very soft and allow a guidewire to be passed through them; balloon dilatation alone can then be effectively utilized. Also, even if the guidewire does not pass, the laser can still be used to adequately recanalize a short segment. Many new types of lasers are now being tried (e.g., excimer lasers). In our opinion, however, regardless of the laser type utilized, it is in such short segments that the principle of LABA may most effectively be applied.

For those reasons, though we realize that balloon dilatation and LABA are not universally applicable, it is premature to abandon this technique. As long-term data became available, it may eventually be possible to eliminate the balloon dilator competely and replace it with sequential laser disobstruction. This would avoid the attendant complications of balloon dilatation. Furthermore, other currently available adjunctive procedures are not practical in all situations. Atherectomy is very popular at present, but it simply takes too long to perform for it to replace LABA as an adjunct to bypass surgery. Furthermore, it is only acceptable for tight stenoses. Totally obstructed lesions still require laser disobstruction.

Ultimately, the key to the success of any procedure is its durability. Long-term data with respect to LABA are still accumulating. Therefore, it should remain a technique to be learned and applied by vascular surgeons in selected situations. There is no ideal vascular procedure at present. Laser-assisted balloon angioplasty, like many other procedures, must with time find its appropriate niche in the surgeon's armamentarium.

REFERENCES

1. Einstein A. Zur Quantentheorie der Strahlung. *Phisiol Z.* 18:121-128, 1917.
2. Schawlow AL, Townes CH. Infrared and optical lasers. *Phys Rev.* 112:1940, 1958.
3. Maiman TH. Stimulated optical radiation in ruby. *Nature.* 187:493-494, 1960.
4. Campbell CJ, Rittler MC, Koester CJ. The optical laser as a retinal coagulation: An evaluation. *Trans Am Acad Ophthalmol Otolaryngol.* 67:58, 1963.
5. L'Esperance FA Jr. *Ophthalmic Lasers: Photocoagulation, Photoradiation and Surgery.* CV Mosby, St. Louis, 1983.
6. Diabetic Retinopathy Study Research Group. Photocoagulation treatment of proliferative diabetic retinopathy. *Ophthalmology.* 88:583-600, 1981.
7. Cruess AF, Stephens KF, Magargal LE, Brown GC. Peripheral circumferential retinal scatter photocoagulation for treatment of proliferative sickle retinopathy. *Ophthalmology.* 90:272-278, 1983.
8. Branch Vein Occlusion Study Group. Argon laser photocoagulation for macular edema in branch vein occlusion. *Am J Ophthalmol.* 98:271-282, 1984.
9. Beamis JF Jr, Shapshay SM. Nd:YAG laser therapy for tracheobronchial disorders. *Head Neck Surg.* 75:173-180, 1984.
10. Strong MS. Laser excision of carcinoma of the larynx, *Laryngoscope.* 85:1286-1289. 1975.
11. Andrews AH, Horowitz SL. Bronchoscopic CO_2 laser surgery. *Lasers Surg Med.* 1:35-45, 1980.
12. Balchum OT, Doiron DR. Photoradiation therapy of endobronchial lung cancer. *Clin Chest Med.* 6:255-275, 1985.
13. Casey LR, Fairfax WR, Smith SJ, Dixon JA. Intratracheal fire ignited by the Nd:YAG laser during treatment of tracheal stenosis. *Chest.* 84:295-296, 1983.
14. Strong MS, Vaughan CW, Jako GJ, Polanyi T. Transoral resection of cancer of the oral cavity: The role of the CO_2 Laser. *Otolaryngol Clin North Am.* 12:207-218, 1979.
15. Mittelman H. CO_2 laser turbinectomies for chronic obstructive rhinitis. *Lasers Surg Med.* 2:29-36, 1982.
16. DeSanto LW. The options in early laryngeal carcinoma. *N Engl J Med.* 4ed 306:910-912, 1982.
17. Hayata Y, Kato H, Konaka C, Ono J, Takizawa N. Hematoporphyrin derivative and laser photoradiation in the treatment of lung cancer. *Chest.* 81:269-277, 1982.
18. Kaplan I, Goldman J, Ger R. The treatment of erosions of the uterine cervix by means of the CO_2 laser. *Obstet Gynecol.* 41:795-796, 1973.
19. Larsson G, Alm P, Grundsell H. Laser conization versus cold knife conization. *Surg Gynecol Obstet.* 154:59-61, 1982.
20. Rosomoff HL, Brown J, Carroll F. Effect of laser on carcinoma in man. *JAMA.* 192:167-168, 1965.
21. Fasano VA, Urciuoli R, Ponzio RM. Photocoagulation of cerebral arteriovenous malformations and arterial aneurysms with the neodymium:yttrium-aluminium-garnet or argon laser: preliminary results in twelve patients. *Neurosurgery.* 11:754-760, 1982.

22. Beck OJ. The use of the Nd:YAG and the CO_2 laser in neurosurgery. *Neurosurg Rev.* 3:261-266, 1 980.

23. Jain KK. Lasers in neurosurgery: A review. *Lasers Surg Med.* 2:217-230, 1983.

24. Fidler JP, Hoefer RW, Polanyi TG, et al. Laser surgery in exsanguinating liver injury. *Ann Surg.* 181:74-80, 1975.

25. Dixon JA, Mliller F, McCloskey D, Siddoway J. Anatomy and techniques in segmental splenectomy. *Surg Gynecol Obstet.* 150:516-520, 1980.

26. Mulvaney WP, Beck CR. The laser beam in urology. *J Urol.* 99:112-115, 1968.

27. Smith JA, Dixon JA. Argon laser phototherapy of superficial transitional cell carcinoma of the bladder. *J Urol.* 131:655-656, 1984.

28. Strong MS, Vaughan CW, Jako GJ, Polanyi T. Transoral resection of cancer of the oral cavity: The role of the CO_2 Laser. *Otolaryngol Clin North Am.* 12:207-218, 1979.

29. DeSanto LW. Selection of treatment for in situ and early invasive carcinoma of the glottis, *Can J Otolaryngol.* 3:552-556, 1974.

30. Strong MS. Laser excision of carcinoma of the larynx. *Laryngoscope.* 85:1286-1289, 1975.

31. McDougall JC, Cortese DA. Neodymium-YAG laser therapy of malignant airway obstruction. *Mayo Clin Proc.* 58:35-39, 1983.

32. Shapshay SM, Dumon JF, Beamis JF Jr. Endoscopic treatment of tracheobronchial malignancy: Experience with Nd-YAG and CO_2 lasers in 506 operations. *Otolaryngol Head Neck Surg.* 93:205-210, 1985.

33. Bellina JH, Ross LF, Voros JI. Colposcopy and the CO_2 laser for treatment of cervical intraepithelial neoplasia: An analysis of seven years' experience. *J Rep Med.* 28:147-151, 1983.

34. Anderson MC. Treatment of cervical intraepithelial neoplasia with the CO_2 laser: Report of 543 patients. *Obstet Gynecol.* 59:720-725, 1982.

35. Burke L. The use of the carbon dioxide laser in the therapy of cervical intraepithelial neoplasia. *Am J Obstet Gynecol.* 144: 337-340, 1982.

36. Benedet JL, Nickerson KG, White GW. Laser therapy for cervical intraepithelial neoplasia. *Obstet Gynecol.* 58:188-191, 1981.

37. Bagsish MS. Management of cervical intraepithelial neoplasia by carbon dioxide laser. *Obstet Gynecol.* 60:378-384, 1982.

38. Townsend DE, Levine RU, Crum DP, Richart RM. Treatment of vaginal carcinoma in situ with the carbon dioxide laser. *Am J Obstet Gynecol.* 143:565-568, 1982.

39. Simonsen E, Johnsson JE, Trope C. CO_2 laser for the treatment of invasive vulvar and vaginal cancer. *Neoplasia.* 30:359, 1983.

40. Dougherty TJ, Kaufman JE, Goldfarb A, et al. Photoradiation therapy for the treatment of malignant tumors. *Cancer Res.* 38:2628-2635, 1978.

41. Ward BG, Forbes IJ, Cowled PA, et al. The treatment of vaginal recurrences of gynecologic malignancy with phototherapy following hematoporphyrin derivative pretreatment. *Am J Obstet Gynecol.* 142:356-357, 1982.

42. Kelly PJ, Alker GJ, Goerss S. Computer assisted stereotactic laser microsurgery for the treatment of intracranial neoplasms. *Neurosurgery.* 10:324-331, 1982.

43. Bartal AD, Heilbronn YD, Auram J, et al. Carbon dioxide laser surgery of basal meningiomas. *Surg Neurol.* 17:90-95, 1982.

44. Strait TA, Robertson JH, Clark WC. Use of the carbon dioxide laser in the operative management of intracranial meningiomas: A report of twenty cases. *Neurosurgery.* 10:464-467, 1982.

45. Robertson JH, Clark WC, Robertson JT, et al. Use of the carbon dioxide laser for acoustic tumor surgery. *Neurosurgery.* 12:286-290, 1983.

46. Beck OJ, Frank F. The use of the Nd:YAG laser in neurosurgery. *Lasers Surg Med.* 5:345-356, 1985.

47. Brunner R, Landthaler M, Haina D, et al. Treatment of benign, semimalignant, and malignant skin tumors with the Nd:YAG laser. *Lasers Surg Med.* 5:105-111, 1985.

48. Dougherty TJ. Photoradiation therapy for cutaneous and subcutaneous malignancies. *J Invest Dermatol.* 77:122-124, 1981.

49. Benson RC, Kinsey JH, Cortese DA, et al. Treatment of transitional cell carcinoma of the bladder with hematoporphyrin derivative phototherapy. *J Urol.* 130:1090-1095, 1983.

50. Moan J, Christensen T, Sommer S. The main photosensitizing components of hematoporphyrin derivative. *Cancer Lett.* 55:161-166, 1982.

51. Rettenmaier MA, Berman ML, DiSaia PJ, et al. Photoradiation therapy of gynecologic malignancies. *Gynecol Oncol.* 17:200-206, 1984.

52. Tsuchiya A, Obara N, Makoto M, et al. Hematoporphyrin derivative and laser photoradiation in the diagnosis and treatment of bladder cancer. *J Urol.* 130:79-82, 1983.

53. Choy DSJ, Stertzer S, Rotterdam H, et al. Laser coronary angioplasty. Experience with nine cadaver hearts. *Am J Cardiol.* 50:1206-1208, 1982.

54. Abela GS, Normann S, Cohen D, et al. Effects of carbon dioxide, Nd:YAG, and argon laser radiation on coronary atheromatous plaques. *Am J Cardiol.* 50:1199-1205, 1982.

55. Lee G, Ikeda RM, Herman I, et al. The qualitative effects of laser irradiation on human arteriosclerotic disease. *Am Heart J.* 105:885-889, 1983.

56. Geschwind H, Boussingnac G, Teisseire B, et al. Percutaneous transluminal laser angioplasty in man. *Lancet.* ii:844, 1984.

57. Ginsburg R, Kim DS, Guthaner D, et al. Salvage of an ischemic limb by laser angioplasty: Description of a new technique. *Clin Cardiol.* 7:54-58, 1984.

58. Choy DS, Stertzer SH, et al. Human coronary laser recanalization. *Clin Cardiol.* 7:377-381, 1984.

59. Ginsburg R, Wexler L, et al. Percutaneous transluminal laser angioplasty for treatment of peripheral vascular disease: Clinical experience with 16 patients. *Radiology.* 156:619-624, 1985.

60. Lee G, Garcia JM, Chan MC, et al. Clinically successful long-term laser coronary recanalization. *Am Heart J.* 112:1323-1325, 1986.

61. Abela GS, Seeger JM, Barbieri E, et al. Laser angioplasty with angioscopic guidance in humans. *J Am Coll Cardiol.* 8:184-192, 1986.

62. Cumberland DC, Tayler DI, et al. Percutaneous laser thermal angioplasty: Initial clinical results with a laser probe in total peripheral artery occlusion. *Lancet.* 1:1457-1459, 1986.

63. Fleisher HL, Thompson BW, McCowan TC, et al. Human percutaneous laser angioplasty. *Am J Surg.* 154:666-670, 1987.

64. Sanborn TA, Greenfield AJ, et al. Human percutaneous and intraoperative laser thermal angioplasty: Initial clinical results as an adjunct to balloon angioplasty. *J Vasc Surg.* 5:83-87, 1987.

65. Matsumoto T, Naide D, Schafer C, et al. Laser angioplasty. *Surg Gynecol Obstet.* 166:81-83, 1988.

66. Matsumoto T, Yang Y, Naide D, et al. Argon laser arterial recanalization. *Pennsylvania Med.* 91:27-30, 1988.

67. Lee G, Masden R, Weiss JA, et al. Percutaneous peripheral laser angioplasty: Demonstration of the clinical safety and efficacy of a new coaxial-guided laser-heated cap system. *Am Heart J.* 116:1640-1641, 1988.

68. Lee G, Argenal AJ, Rink DL, et al. Percutaneous coronary laser angioplasty: Successful clinical application of a new thermal cap catheter coaxially guided over a steerable central guide wire. *Am Heart J.* 116:1637-1638, 1988.

69. Diethrich EB, Timbadia E, Bahadir I, et al. Argon laser-assisted peripheral angioplasty. *Vasc Surg.* 22:77-87, 1988.

70. Matsumoto T, Koyanagi N, Yang Y, DuPree J. Laser arterial recanalization in reconstructive vascular surgery. *Contemporary Surg.* 33:11-19, 1988.

71. Seeger JM, Abela GS, Silverman SH, et al. Initial results of laser recanalization in lower extremity arterial reconstruction. *J Vasc Surg.* 9:10-17, 1989.

72. Matsumoto T, Rajyaguru V, Okamura T. Laser recanalization, laser assisted balloon angioplasty and laser angioplasty. *Surg Gynecol Obstet.* 169:195-198, 1989.

73. Matsumoto T, Okamura T, Rajyaguru V. Laser arterial disobstructive procedures in 148 lower extremities. *J Vasc Surg.* 10:169-177, 1989.

74. Fuller TA, ed. *Surgical Lasers.* Macmillan Publishing Company, New York, 1987.

75. Dixon JA, ed. *Surgical Application of Lasers.* Year Book Medical Publishers Inc., Chicago, 1987.

76. Apfelberg DB, ed. *Evaluation and Installation of Surgical Laser Systems.* Springer-Verlag, New York, 1987.

77. Carruth JAS and Simpson GT, eds. *Laser in Otolaryngology.* Year Book Medical Publishers Inc., Chicago, 1988.

78. Hall RR, Hill DW, Beach AD. A carbon dioxide surgical laser. *Ann Roy Coll Surg.* 48:181-188, 1971.

79. McKenzie AL, Carruth AS. Lasers in surgery and medicine. *Phys Mæed Bio.*l 29:619641, 1984.

80. Litwin FiS, Fine S, Klein E, Fine BS. Burn injury after carbon dioxide laser irradiation. *Arch Surg.* 98:212-222, 1969.

81. Little HL, Zweng HC, Peabody RR. Argon laser slit-lamp retinal photocoagulation. *Trans Am Acad Ophthalmol Otolaryngol.* 74:85, 1970.

82. Goldman L, et al. Treatment of port wine marks by an argon laser. *J Dermatol Surg.* 2:385-388, 1976.

83. Apfelberg DB, Master MR, Lash H. Treatment of Nevi aranei by means of an argon laser. *J Dermatol Surg Oncol.* 4:172-174, 1978.

84. Parkin JL, Dixon JA. Laser phototherapy in hereditary hemorrhagic teleangiectasia. *Otolaryngol Head Neck Surg.* 89:204-208, 1981.

85. Apfelberg DB, Master MR, Lash H, Rivers J. The argon laser for cutaneous lesions. *JAMA.* 245:2073-2075, 1981.

86. Fuller T. Fundamentals of lasers in surgery and medicine. In Dixon JA, ed. *Surgical Applications of Lasers.* Year Book, Chicago, 1987;16-33.

87. Kiefhaber P, Nath G, Moritz K. Endoscopic control of gastrointestinal hemorrhage by irradiation with the high-power neodymium YAG laser. *Prog Surg.* 15:140-155, 1977.

88. Fleischer D. Nd:YAG laser therapy for active variceal bleeding. *Gastroenterology.* 82:1058, 1982.

89. Halpin A, et al. Nd:YAG laser in treatment of serious ill patients with gastrointestinal bleeding. *Gastrintest Endosc.* 33:199-202, 1987.

90. Brunetaud JM, Maunoury V, Ducrotte P, et al. Palliative treatment of rectosigmoid carcinoma by laser endoscopic photoablation. *Gastroenterology.* 92:663-668, 1987.

91. Schroder T, Brackett K, Joffe SN. Proximal pancreatectomy: A comparison of electrocautery and contact and noncontact Nd:YAG laser techniques in dog. *Am J Surg.* 154:493-498, 1987.

92. Dixon JA. Current laser applications in general surgery. *Ann Surg.* 207:355-372, 1988.

93. Jensen DM, Machicado G, Randall G, et al. Comparison of low-power YAG laser and BICAP tumor probe for palliation of esophageal cancer strictures. *Gastroenterology.* 94:1263-1270, 1988.

94. Cross FW, Bowker TJ. The physical properties of tissue ablation with excimer lasers. *Med Instrumentation.* 21:226-230, 1987.

95. Isner JM, Donaldson RF, Deckelbaum LI, et al. The excimer laser: gross, light microscopic and ultrastructural analysis of potential advantages for use in laser therapy of cardiovascular disease. *J Am Coll Cardiol.* 6:1102-1109, 1985.

96. Forrester JS. Laser angioplasty. Now and in the future. *Circulation.* 78:777-779, 1988.

97. Sliney D, Wolbarsht M. *Safety with lasers and other optical sources.* Plenum Press, New York, 1980.

98. Beatrice ES, Randolph DI, Stuck BE, Lund DJ. Laser hazards: Biomedical threshold level investigations. *Milit Med.* 142:889-892, 1977.

99. Solon LK. Occupational safety with laser (optical maser) beams. *Arch Environ H.* 6:414, 1963.

100. Powell CH, Goldman L. Recommendations of the Laser Safety Conference. *Arch Environ H.* 18:448, 1969.

101. American National Standards Institute. *Safe Use of Lasers.* ANSI Standard Z136.1, New York, 1973.

102. American Conference of Governmental Industrial Hygienists. *A Guide for Control of Laser Hazards.* ACGIH, Cincinnati, 1973.

103. Bauman N. Angioplasty lasers may zap heart attacks in 1990. *Laser Med Surg News Advances.* 6:1-6, 1989.

Appendix

Guidelines for Laser Use, Maintenance and Education at the Hahnemann University Hospital

POLICY: To ensure the proper use of lasers, delivery systems and equipment.

PURPOSE: A. To provide for patient and personnel safety during laser use.

B. To provide for proper care and maintenance of lasers.

SCOPE: This policy is observed by all surgeons, anesthesiologists, nurses and technical personnel.

IMPLEMENTATION: This policy is implemented by the Laser Safety Committee.

PROCEDURE:

A. Patient Safety

1. Only credentialed/approved physicians shall be permitted laser use. Credentialing shall be maintained by the Laser Safety Committee.
2. The surgeon shall assume responsibility for selecting the laser type, wattage, mode and delivery system for each procedure.
3. To minimize the possibility of fire, the laser shall not be used in conjunction with alcohol, ether, benzoin or combustible anesthetic gases. Water must be readily available in the event of a fire.
4. The anesthesiologist shall protect the endotracheal tube from the laser beam whenever the two are in close proximity. Non-flammable tubes or specially wrapped tubes shall be used to minimize the possibility of a fire.
5. Protect the surrounding tissues from potential damage resulting from reflected laser energy and heat by:
   a. covering the tissue with wet sponges, laps, cottonoids and/or towels.
   b. irrigating the surrounding tissue area to decrease the temperature.
   c. using non-reflective alignment of the eye and laser beam.
6. Protectively cover the patient's eyes with pads (when asleep) or with appropriate wavelength glasses (when awake) whenever possible direct or reflective alignment of the eye and laser beam exists.
7. When the laser is being used in close proximity to the rectum, the orifice shall be packed with a wet sponge or packing and/or covered with moist towels. (Methane rectal gas is flammable.)
8. The Laser Nurse is responsible for completintg and maintaining a laser log and safety checklist on all procedures (see attached).
9. When the unit is not in use, the laser is to be placed on "stand by" or when available, the beam shutter is to be closed in an effort to avoid accidental discharge toward an area not involved in the surgery or toward OR personnel. The laser shall not be left unattended at anytime during the procedure.
10. The key to the laser is to be accessible only to persons approved for use of the laser. Under no circumstances is the key to be maintained in the laser.

    *Solutions used for patient skin preps should contain no free alcohol. If alcohol is present extreme care must be taken to allow time for evaporation/drying. Side/drip towels must also be used to prevent pooling of prep solutions. These must be removed before patient draping. Approved solutions available include povidone, iodine and chlorhexidine.

B. Personnel Safety

1. All nursing personnel working with lasers shall be credentialed by the Laser Safety Officers (LSO).
2. All personnel in the room shall wear appropriate protective eyewear.
3. Baseline, periodic and exit eye exams shall be conducted on all appropriate personnel.
4. A standard laser danger sign (ANSI approved) shall be posted on all entrances to the OR where the laser is to be used.
5. The operator's manual shall be attached to the cabinet of the laser and shall be available to all personnel operating the laser.
6. Injuries resulting from the laser shall be reported immediately to the person in charge. Incident reports shall be completed as soon as possible following the incident.
7. To prevent accidents, the laser beam shall not be directed at any person other than the patient's operative site.
8. To avoid accidental discharge of the laser, only the user physician shall have access to the laser foot pedal. Other foot pedals (eg. bipolar) shall be operated by the surgical assistant.
9. Only necessary personnel are permitted in the OR during laser use.
10. The laser produces a non-ionizing form of electromagnetic radiation and is therefore *not* a threat to an unborn fetus.
11. A smoke evacuation system designed for plume removal shall be used during laser procedures, as appropriate.

C. Proper Care of the Laser

1. Only qualified and trained employees shall be assigned to install, adjust and operate the laser equipment.
2. Removable laser parts shall be stored in a place accessible only to qualified and trained employees.
3. A Laser Nurse who has been trained in laser use shall be assigned to all cases.
4. When technical difficulties arise with the laser unit that are beyond the realm of the Laser Nurse, the Biomedical Engineering Department shall be called. *Any* malfunction of the laser unit must be reported to the Biomedical Engineering Department.

D. Personnel Education

1. An RN (or private laser technician) educated/credentialed on laser use, shall be assigned to monitor, control the laser, enforce safety guidelines and document the use for each laser procedure.
2. RN credentialing includes:
   a. Attendance at the house course offered by the LSO.
   b. Demonstration of "Hands-On" knowledge to the LSO.
   c. Operate the laser during two (2) procedures (2 times for each laser type) in conjunction with the Clinical LSO.
   d. Yearly laser update (seminar, review course, etc.).

LASER DELIVERY SYSTEMS/EQUIPMENT

ADDENDUM

Nd:YAG

#90-6065 Surgi-light GU disposable fiberoptic delivery system

Argon

HGM Endocoagulator Model 5 Laser

HGM Fleischman-Swartz endo-ocular probe (st & angle) delivery system

Safety goggles: 450-532 nm (5 pr.) OD 5 @ 488/514.5 nm

#S-060 HGM micro surgery filter for *Wild* scope

Warning signs